DATE DUE

DEMCO, INC. 38-2931

Differe
Surgic   nent
and

Differentiating Surgical Equipment and Supplies

Colleen J. Rutherford, RN, MSN, CNOR
Educator
Concord Hospital
Concord, New Hampshire

F.A. Davis Company • Philadelphia

F. A. Davis Company
1915 Arch Street
Philadelphia, PA 19103
www.fadavis.com

Copyright © 2010 by F. A. Davis Company

Printed in the United States of America

Last digit indicates print number: 10 9 8 7 6 5 4 3 2 1

Acquisitions Editor: Christa Fratantoro
Developmental Editor: Yvonne Gillam
Publisher: Margaret Biblis
Manager of Content Development: George W. Lang
Art and Design Manager: Carolyn O'Brien

As new scientific information becomes available through basic and clinical research, recommended treatments and drug therapies undergo changes. The author(s) and publisher have done everything possible to make this book accurate, up to date, and in accord with accepted standards at the time of publication. The author(s), editors, and publisher are not responsible for errors or omissions or for consequences from application of the book, and make no warranty, expressed or implied, in regard to the contents of the book. Any practice described in this book should be applied by the reader in accordance with professional standards of care used in regard to the unique circumstances that may apply in each situation. The reader is advised always to check product information (package inserts) for changes and new information regarding dose and contraindications before administering any drug. Caution is especially urged when using new or infrequently ordered drugs.

Library of Congress Cataloging-in-Publication Data

Rutherford, Colleen.
   Differentiating surgical equipment and supplies / Colleen J. Rutherford.
     p. ; cm.
   Includes index.
   ISBN 978-0-8036-1572-4
1. Surgery—Equipment and supplies—Handbooks, manuals, etc. I. Title.
   [DNLM: 1. Surgical Equipment—Atlases. 2. Equipment and Supplies—Atlases.
3. Operating Rooms—organization & administration—Atlases. WO 517 R975d 2009]
   RD32.R695 2009
   617.9—dc22
                                                   2009023553

Acknowledgements

No one writes a book alone. I would like to acknowledge the following people and resources for their contributions to this project:

First, to Christa Fratantoro, Acquisitions Editor of F.A. Davis Publishing Company—you had enough faith in me to let me write a second book. Yvonne Gillam, Developmental Editor of F. A. Davis Publishing Company—your energy and enthusiasm toward this project helped to make it happen. Both of you make writing a pleasure and keep me motivated. I cherish you as business associates and friends.

To Jamie—Thanks for your patience and perseverance in taking the photos for this book. You are a true artist.

To my mother—Thank you for the love and support you have given me throughout my life. I would not be the person I am today without your love and caring.

To all of my friends—you continue to enrich my life on a daily basis. I am truly blessed to have each and every one of you in my life. To Marie DeRosia—you are a wonderful friend and terrific colleague. Thank you for your support and your willingness to "model" for some of the photos in this book—what a true friend!

A special "thank you" to Sharon Guldin, CRNA, Sean O'Brien, CRNA, and Robert Sanborn, CRNA, for their careful review and input regarding the anesthesia content.

I have used numerous websites and surgical equipment catalogs to double check facts and information on the equipment and supplies in this book.

Reviewers

David A. Alfaro, CST
Program Director
American Career College
Surgical Technology Department
Los Angeles, California

Christina Lynn Baumer, RN, PhD, MEd, CNOR, CHES
Chair
Division of Continuing Education
Program Director
Surgical Technology
Lancaster General College of Nursing and Health Sciences
Continuing Education
Surgical Technology
Lancaster, Pennsylvania

Karen L. Chambers, CST-ACLS
Director
Long Island University
Surgical Technology Institute
School of Continuing Studies
Brooklyn, New York

Kevin R. Craycraft, CST
Program Director
Bluegrass Community and Technical College
Health and Human Services Department
Lexington, Kentucky

Javier E. Espinales, MEd, CST
Director, Surgical Technology Program
Virginia College at Austin
Surgical Technology Department
Austin, Texas

Robin Hueske, CST
Concorde Career Institute
Surgical Technology Department
Aurora, Colorado

Tammy Mangold, MEd, CST, CFA
Surgical Technologist
Columbia Regional Hospital
Surgery Department
Colombia, Missouri

Diane May, CST
Associate Professor
Santa Fe Community College
Health Sciences Division
Gainesville, Florida

Rosemary A. Nagler, RN, BS, CNOR
Clinical Education Coordinator
Western Suffolk BOCES
School of Surgical Technology
Northport, New York

Judith Schatte, RN, CNOR, CRNFA
Program Director and Instructor
Surgical Technology
Brevard Community College
Cocoa, Florida

Deborah S. Smith, RN, CNOR
Director and Instructor
Southeastern Technical College
Surgical Technology Department
Glenwood, Georgia

Roy G. Zacharias, Jr, BS, CST
Associate Academic Dean
Concorde Career Institute
Surgical Technology Department
Arlington, Texas

Table of Contents

Introduction

Entering the operating room for the first time can be intimidating; it is like entering a foreign land. The clothes are different (scrubs, masks and hats), the temperature cold and there are lots of equipment and supplies that are not used anywhere else except in surgery. What is a "lap pad"? What is the difference between "Chromic" and "Vicryl" suture? What safety precautions are necessary when the laser is in use? This book answers those questions and a whole lot more.

The purpose of this book is to lessen the intimidation by describing common equipment and supplies unique to the surgical setting. Throughout the chapters there are special pages that describe some equipment or supplies in detail, help differentiate between similar supplies (e.g., types of suture), aid in troubleshooting equipment or, in the case of anesthesia, give the reader key points to look for when aiding in patient care. In some cases, the equipment and supplies require less narration; on those pages you will find pictures of the supply and a short description, including its use.

Throughout the chapters you will find boxes titled "Watch Out!" The purpose of these boxes is to draw your attention to important information.

Students and new personnel can use the book as a reference, look up supplies and equipment that they have come across in surgical cases or read more information about a subject. Instructors and preceptors can use the book as a learning aid, assigning personnel or students certain chapters to read or items to look up. Instructors who adopt this book for use in their classrooms also receive a CD-ROM containing test questions and pictures of the supplies and equipment that can be inserted into their own tests or presentations.

The operating room is an exciting and wonderful foreign land, full of joys and some sorrows but most of all wonderful opportunities to learn and make a difference for others. It is my hope that you find this book a valuable aid in navigating the exciting world of surgery!

CHAPTER 1

Common Equipment and Furniture

ASEPTIC (STERILE) TECHNIQUE

Aseptic technique is the foundation of all that goes on in the operating room (OR). No matter what else happens, failure to practice proper aseptic technique increases the patient's risk of infection, injury or even death.

Asepsis literally means "without infection," but the generally accepted definition is "absence of all microbes." In surgery, an inanimate object (e.g., instrument or supply) is considered sterile (aseptic) only after it has been exposed to a process that kills all microbes, including spores. Sterilization processes can use steam, gas, chemicals, hydrogen peroxide or radiation to render an item free of microbes. The skin can never be rendered *sterile* (i.e., free of all microbes); therefore, aseptic technique dealing with skin (e.g., scrubbing or prepping) is aimed at reducing microbes to an absolute minimum.

This section of the book covers principles of aseptic technique and provides an overview of sterilization methods. It is imperative that ALL personnel working in the OR have a thorough understanding of aseptic technique in order to protect their patients.

> **WATCH OUT!** **Surgical Conscience**
>
> - *Surgical conscience* is the ethical motivation to practice proper aseptic technique. ALL personnel must be willing to police themselves and each other, be willing to admit to a break in technique and be ready to take corrective action. The willingness to police oneself, whether or not there is anyone else around to notice the break in technique, is imperative. Anyone who is not willing to admit to a break in technique should NOT be working in the OR.
>
> - ANY break in sterile technique, no matter how minor it may seem, puts the patient at increased risk of infection.
>
> - There is no such thing as "slightly contaminated" or "almost sterile." Sterility of an item is an absolute—either an item is sterile or it is not. If there is ANY doubt about an item's sterility, DO NOT use it—dispose of it and get a new one.

Principles and Guidelines of Aseptic Technique

The principles listed here are adapted from various OR textbooks as well as the Association of Operating Room Nurses (AORN) guidelines and standards of practice. Although some of these principles and guidelines may be practiced and enforced to varying degrees, depending on institutional policies, they have a solid foundation in patient care and safety.

- Only sterile (scrubbed) personnel handle sterile items. Only nonsterile personnel handle nonsterile items.

- Sterility of an item is an absolute—either an item is sterile or it is not. If there is ANY doubt about an item's sterility, DO NOT use it—dispose of it and get a new one.

- Proper attire must be worn by all personnel. This includes scrub suits, masks covering the mouth and nose, hats or caps that cover all hair (including facial hair) and, in some cases, eye protection and shoe covers. Waist ties and scrub tops should be tucked inside the pants to prevent inadvertent contamination of the field. Long sleeved jackets may be worn by nonsterile personnel but need to be buttoned.

- The wearing of cloth hats or caps depends on institutional policy. Cloth caps should be thrown into the laundry at the end of the day and when they become visibly soiled. Cloth hats that are worn for more than 1 day without being laundered become a source of increased microbial contamination.

- Jewelry is a potential source of microbes and should NOT be worn in the OR.

- Nonsterile persons must stand a *minimum* of 12 to 18 inches away from any sterile area (e.g., the sterile field, sterile tables or ring basins). Nonsterile items should be kept a minimum of 12 inches away from sterile items.

- The draped patient is the center of the sterile field, and all other components of the sterile field (e.g., Mayo stand, back tables and ring stand) should be placed close to and around the patient. Nonsterile items or personnel should not be within this area.

- The sterile field should be created as close to the time of surgery as possible. The longer sterile items are left out, the greater the chance of contamination. Rooms with sterile items left open for more than 1 to 2 hours (this time varies depending on institutional policy but 2 hours is the maximum allowable time) should be broken down and the items removed.

- If sterile items are opened in a room and the surgery starting time is delayed, the room must be continuously monitored. It is NOT acceptable to leave the room without someone there to monitor it at all times. If the room is left unattended there is no way to tell if an item or items might have been inadvertently contaminated.

- Talking at the sterile field should be kept to a minimum. Excessive, non-essential talking increases the amount of airborne microbes.

- Movement (including traffic in and out of the room) should be kept to a minimum during the surgical procedure. Doors should be kept closed. Opening of doors and movement of personnel stir up air currents that can lead to increased microbial contamination.

Continued

Principles and Guidelines of Aseptic Technique—cont'd

■ Handling and moving drapes and linen should be kept to a minimum to prevent the spread of lint and dust.

■ The only part of the surgical table that is considered sterile is the TABLETOP. Sterile items should NOT hang over the table edge.

■ Once placed, table drapes and patient drapes should be left in place. Repositioning drapes could cause a part of the drape that previously had been below tabletop or patient level (therefore unsterile) to be brought back into the sterile field.

■ Tubing that falls below the level of the patient is considered contaminated. If the electrosurgical hand unit or suction tip falls below the patient level it must be discarded and replaced with a new one.

■ The only parts of the sterile gown that are considered sterile are the front of the gown from waist up to mid-chest and the sleeves to 2 inches above the elbow (see Fig. 1-1). The stockinette cuffs are NOT considered sterile because they are not impervious to perspiration, which can wick upward through the stockinette, bringing microbes with it.

■ Scrubbed personnel should NOT place their hands in their axillary (armpit) area. Even though scrubbed personnel are wearing sterile gowns, strike through contamination could occur from perspiration wicking from the high microbial count in the axillary area.

■ Only an item that has been processed using an approved method is considered sterile. Check sterilization indicators on all items to make sure they have been exposed to the proper conditions to render them sterile.

■ Prior to introducing an item into the sterile field, inspect it for any breaks in the integrity of the wrapper (see Fig. 1-2). If the wrapper has a hole (no matter how small), a tear or a break in the integrity of the seal or if the wrapper is wet or the sterilization indicator is missing or has not turned color, the item is NOT considered sterile and CANNOT be used.

■ Store sterile items in a clean, dry area. Sterile items should NOT be stored in a dirty work area or with unsterile items. They should NOT be stored under sinks or anywhere there is a possibility of being exposed to moisture.

■ Once scrubbed and properly attired, sterile personnel should remain within the immediate area of the sterile field. Sterile personnel should NOT leave the sterile field or the room to retrieve items; needed items should be brought to them by nonsterile personnel. The further sterile personnel move away from the sterile field, the greater the chance of contamination.

■ If sterile personnel must change positions during the procedure, they must move around each other either by moving front to front or back to back. The unsterile back of one person's gown should NOT be facing the sterile front of the other person.

■ Nonsterile personnel should NOT walk between two sterile surfaces (e.g., the circulating nurse should not walk between two sterile tables that are next to each other).

■ Nonsterile personnel should NOT reach over the sterile field to deliver an item to the sterile field. The item should be flipped onto the field from the package or the open package presented to the scrub person so that he or she can retrieve the item without contamination.

■ When pouring solutions into basins on the sterile field, the nonsterile person should pour slowly to minimize splash onto the sterile field. Unless the drape is impervious, moisture can draw microbes up from the unsterile surface (it acts as a "wick"). This is known as *strike through* contamination.

■ Basins, graduates or medication cups should be held outward by the scrub person or placed at the edge of the table (see Fig. 1-3) to receive fluids or medication. This allows the nonsterile person to pour the solution without reaching over the field.

■ Materials used for drapes and barriers should be strong, moisture resistant and low linting.

■ A 1-inch margin around the edge of a sterile wrapper or covering is considered unsterile. Care must be taken not to allow a sterile item to drag over the edge of wrapper when distributing it to the sterile field (see Fig. 1-4).

■ When opening a sterile package, the nonsterile person should protect his or her hand underneath the wrapper to avoid having it contact the sterile item.

FIGURE 1-1 Areas of the gown considered sterile.

FIGURE 1-2 These items should NOT be used.

FIGURE 1-3 Place graduate and medicine cup near the edge of the table.

FIGURE 1-4 A 1-inch margin around the perimeter is considered to be NOT sterile.

- When retrieving a sterile item from a package, the scrub person should reach straight into the package and pull the item straight upward out of the package, making sure not to touch the item on the unsterile edge of the wrapper.
- All personal protective equipment (e.g., gowns, gloves and masks) should be properly removed at the end of the case and discarded.
- All sharps must be discarded into a puncture-proof sharps bucket in the OR at the end of the case. Sharps should NOT be transported to the dirty work room to be disposed of as transporting increases the chance that someone could get stuck or injured.
- At the beginning of the day and between each case, all furniture surfaces (including lights, tables, bed and so on) are cleaned with a disinfectant and the floor mopped according to institutional policy. Bed padding should be lifted up and cleaned underneath if there is ANY chance that blood or body fluid may have gotten under it.

Opening Sterile Supplies

Opening supplies and distributing them to the sterile field is not difficult to learn, but it does require some practice. It also requires vigilance on the part of the entire surgical team. As stated previously, there is NO compromise to sterile technique. If any item is contaminated (no matter how "minor" the contamination may seem), it must be discard and replaced with a new one. Failure to follow strict standards of asepsis places the patient at risk!

Opening a Pack Onto a Table

The large pack (also known as a *trace pack* or a *case pack*) is the first thing opened when you are preparing a room for surgery (see Fig. 1-5). Opening the large pack(s) first creates a sterile field(s) on which other sterile items can be distributed.

Prior to placing the large pack on the table, the outer plastic cover (i.e., dust cover) should be inspected for any tears or holes. If there are *any* tears or holes DO NOT use the pack; get another one. Once the dust cover has been inspected, remove it and inspect the outer wrapping of the pack (see Fig. 1-6). Again, if there are any holes or tears, DO NOT use it. To open a large pack, place it in the center of the table (it should have a label that says which side of the pack faces the back of the table).

Break the seal on the pack (*Warning:* If the seal is broken when the pack is taken out of the dust cover, DO NOT use it; the seal should be intact until you break it.) and fold

the long ends of the pack outward to cover the table (see Figs. 1-7 and 1-8).

Unfold the layers outward so that they cover the entire surface of the table. Remember: Handle the layers by their edges and pull the layers toward you so that you are not reaching over the sterile area (see Fig. 1-9). Once the pack has been unfolded onto the table, DO NOT readjust it; only the tabletop is considered sterile, and readjusting it will bring a part of the drape that has been below tabletop level (therefore unsterile) up into the sterile field.

FIGURE 1-5 Large pack.

Opening a Peel-Pouched Item

Many sterile items come in a peel-pouch. The item is placed in a pouch, the edges are sealed and the item put through sterile processing. The edges are sealed in such a way that when a person grabs one side of the top in each hand and pulls outward in opposing directions, the pouch peels apart, making it easy to access the item inside (see Fig. 1-10).

Peel-pouch items that are small (e.g., sutures and peanut sponges) can be opened and distributed to the sterile field by "flipping" them onto the field. Items that are large, awkward or potentially could puncture the sterile drape if flipped onto the field (e.g., instruments) should be opened and presented to the scrub person for him or her to take from the package (see Fig. 1-11).

FIGURE 1–6 Pack in the middle of an instrument table.

FIGURE 1–9 A) and B) Edge layers of the pack being unfolded. Remember to unfold the pack toward your body.

FIGURE 1–7 Pack with one end unfolded.

FIGURE 1–8 Pack on the table with both ends unfolded.

FIGURE 1–10 Two peel-pouched items.

FIGURE 1–11 A) Item is being "flipped" onto the sterile field. B) The sterile package opened and presented to the scrub person taking the item.

FIGURE 1–12 A) Hand grasping an envelope-style wrapped package. B) An envelope-style package on a small table.

Opening an Envelope-Style Package

Items that come wrapped in an envelope-style package include linens, some drapes, gowns, basin sets and some individual instruments or small instrument sets. To open this type of package, you need first to grasp the package in one hand so that the flap furthest from you is opened first.

Note: These same steps can be used to open an envelope-wrapped instrument tray on a small table. Instead of grasping the tray in your hand, set it on the table with the first flap to be opened furthest away from you (see Fig. 1-12). This same method is used to open the basin set into the ring stand and follow the same steps.

Open the flap furthest away from you first. Pull the flap downward and away from the sterile item. If you are holding the item, secure this flap by holding it in your hand underneath the package (see Fig. 1-13).

Open each of the side flaps by pulling them out and downward away from the sterile item (see Figs. 1-14 and 1-15).

Open the flap closest to the body last. Pull the flap toward your body and downward, securing it so that it does not flap back and contaminate the item (see Fig. 1-16). If you are holding the item, it can now either be flipped into the sterile field or presented to the scrubbed person for them to take. If the item is on a table, the tabletop is now

FIGURE 1–13 A) Hand holding an item with first flap unfolded and secured. B) Item on a table with the first flap unfolded.

FIGURE 1–14 A) Hand opens side flap keeping the open side flap secure. B) Second flap opened and covering the edge of the table.

covered by the inside of the wrapper and is considered a sterile field. Care needs to be taken not to contaminate the tabletop.

Opening a Genesis Instrument Pan

Some institutions assemble and sterilize their larger instruments sets inside a Genesis instrument pan. Before opening the instrument pan, look at both sides of the instrument pan to determine the location of the handles used to open it. There should be a plastic arrow with an indicator on it inserted through a hole in the handle system (see Fig. 1–17). This ensures that the arrow will be broken when the pan is opened. DO NOT use the instruments set if *either* of the arrows is missing or broken or if the indicator has not turned black.

Look at the top of the pan to make sure you can see a filter showing through the holes in the top of the lid. If the filter is missing, DO NOT use the instrument set.

If both arrows are present and unbroken, the indicators are black and the filter is present in the lid, insert your fingers under the handles and lift upward to break the seal and remove the lid. Remove the lid by lifting straight up and then away from the instrument pan. DO NOT reach over the inside of the pan. Once the lid has been removed, take the filter out of the lid of the tray and inspect it to make sure there are not any holes in it or that

FIGURE 1–15 Item on a table with three flaps open (the furthest one and both side flaps)

it is not wet. If the filter is wet or has holes, DO NOT use the instrument set.

Look at the instrument tray inside the pan. There should be a piece of chemical indicator tape inside the tray (see Fig. 1–18). Look at the tape to make sure it has turned color; usually it will have black stripes on it. If the tape is not obvious, the scrubbed person may have to move instruments in the tray to look for it.

FIGURE 1–16 A) Handheld item completely opened. B) Completely open item on table.

FIGURE 1–17 The indicator on the arrow should be black.

FIGURE 1–18 The stripes on the indicator tape should be black.

FIGURE 1–19 Bottom of the pan with a filter in place and the bottom dry.

If the indicator tape is present and has turned the proper color, the scrub person removes the instrument set from the pan by lifting it straight out and away from the pan. The scrub person holds the instrument set until the nonsterile person has a chance to look at the bottom of the pan to make sure that there is a filter present, that the filter is not wet and does not have any holes in it and that the bottom of the pan does not contain water (see Fig. 1-19). Once the nonsterile person is satisfied that the bottom of the pan is dry and the filter intact, the scrub person may place the instrument tray on his or her back table.

Distributing Fluids to the Field

Fluids should only be distributed into a sterile container that is placed close to the edge of the sterile field or held in the hand of the scrub person. The nonsterile person should NOT reach over the sterile field to pour fluid into a container. Fluid should be distributed by pouring the entire container (or desired amount) all at once into the receptacle without stopping. Care should be taken to hold the lip of the container close enough to the receptacle to avoid splashing the fluid on the field but the lip *cannot* be so close as to touch the rim of the receptacle and contaminate it (see Fig. 1-20).

Important: Prior to the distribution of any fluid onto the sterile field, the type and strength of the solution as well as the expiration date MUST be verified by BOTH the person pouring the solution and the scrub person. BOTH parties

FIGURE 1–20 A) Labeled receptacle. B) Saline fluid being distributed into a container.

> **WATCH OUT!** **Sterilization and Bioburden**
>
> - *Bioburden* is any blood, tissue or body fluid (e.g., pus, vomit, feces or skin oil) that could be present on an instrument or item.
>
> - ALL bioburden MUST be removed before placing an item in the sterilizer either to flash it or to send it through a full cycle. Bioburden may be removed by washing all visible contaminants from the instrument as well as by sending the instrument through a washer.
>
> - If you open a tray and there is blood or dirt on an instrument, DO NOT use it! There is NO such thing as "sterile blood" or any other "sterile contaminant!" Sterilants cannot penetrate bioburden; therefore, the area under the bioburden is NOT sterile.

must visualize the label as well as verbally acknowledging what is being poured into the receptacle. The scrub person must then *immediately* label the receptacle with the type and strength of fluid it contains. Unmarked fluids on the sterile field are an *unacceptable* practice because of the potential to harm the patient.

TYPES OF STERILIZATION

All items that are distributed to and used within the sterile field have to undergo a sterilization process prior to being used. There are several different methods available, all of which have the potential to render an item sterile. The method used usually depends on the item that is being sterilized. Steam under pressure is the most common and cost-effective method of sterilization but cannot be used for items that could be damaged by moisture or pressure. This section is an overview of the different types of sterilization processes available and when each type is used.

Steam Sterilization

As just stated, steam sterilization is the most common and economical method of sterilization. Steam by itself is not an

effective sterilization method. The steam must be under pressure for a specific amount of time before it can render an item sterile. The pressure is used to raise the temperature of the steam up to 250°F to 270°F, high enough to kill all microbial life (including spores).

The steam sterilizer is an enclosed chamber that pressurizes the steam to specific levels. The pressure needed to raise the temperature of the steam to 250°F is 15 psig (pounds per square inch gauge). To raise it to 270°F requires a pressure of 27 psig. It is important to note that these settings are for sea level atmospheres. If your institution is located at a higher elevation, the pressure inside the chamber needs to be increased to achieve levels adequate for sterilization. Generally, this means an increase of 0.5 psig for every 1000 feet above sea level.

There are two basic types of steam sterilizers: gravity displacement and prevacuum. In a gravity displacement sterilization chamber, the air is pushed downward (by gravity) and out through a valve by the pressurized steam. All of the air is removed from the chamber, leaving the pressurized steam to sterilize the items. In this type of sterilizer it is important that items be loaded properly because, if items are improperly placed, they can trap air, which will act as an insulator against the steam. Any items in these air pockets will not be sterile. Minimum exposure time (at 250°F) depends on the items in the load and can vary from 15 to 45 minutes or more. These times do not include that needed for the chamber to fill with steam, for the chamber to get up to temperature, and for the chamber to cool down after exposure to the steam. The complete sterilization cycle is longer (about 2 hours), which must be considered in turnaround time for items needed for subsequent cases.

In contrast to the gravity displacement sterilizer, the prevacuum sterilizer does not rely on gravity to remove the air. In the prevacuum sterilizer the air is pulled out of the chamber using a built-in vacuum device. The air is pulled out rather than displaced using gravity; therefore, there is greater steam penetration in a shorter period of time. Prevacuum sterilizers operate at 270°F and the exposure times are much shorter than gravity displacement sterilizers require. The minimum exposure for most items in a prevacuum sterilizer is 3 to 4 minutes. Again, this does not take into account the time for the air to leave the chamber or cool down time at the end; planning ahead is essential for items needed for subsequent cases.

Flash Sterilization

Flash sterilizers are used in the OR to resterilize quickly an item that has become contaminated but is needed to finish the surgical procedure (see Fig. 1-21). This type of sterilization should *only* be used when there is no other alternative. Before flashing an item, make sure there is not another of the same item available that is already sterile (e.g., in a rack or cabinet of peel-pouched items or from central sterile supply). Items that are flash sterilized are unwrapped and *must* be washed (and free of visible bioburden) before placing them in the sterilizer. The item or items should be placed in a pan with a mesh-type bottom to allow for the steam to reach all surfaces. A piece of indicator tape must be placed in the pan with every load. Failure to include the indicator tape means that there will be no visible monitor to indicate that proper sterilization conditions occurred; therefore, the item cannot be used and the cycle would be need to run again.

Flash sterilizers heat the steam to 270°F to 275°F. The minimum exposure time in a gravity displacement flash sterilizer for metal items without a lumen is 3 minutes and 10 minutes for items with a lumen. Minimum exposure times for prevacuum flash sterilizers are 3 minutes for metal items without a lumen and 4 minutes for items with a lumen or those that are porous. Remember the complete cycle is longer, usually 10 to 20 minutes.

FIGURE 1-21 Flash sterilizer.

> **WATCH OUT!**
>
> ## A Few More Considerations for Flash Sterilization
>
> - Cameras, scopes, power equipment or other delicate items should NOT be flashed sterilized unless you have thoroughly read the manufacturer's instructions and found that they indicate it is safe to do so.
> - Implants should NEVER be flashed sterilized. IF you HAVE NO OTHER CHOICE in an *emergency*, a rapid readout biological monitoring device (not a piece of indicator tape) must be placed in the pan with the implant.
> - Flash sterilizers need to be located in an area outside the OR room but close to the doorway so that items can be quickly and directly transported to the sterile field.
> - Items to be flash sterilized are unwrapped unless the manufacturer's instructions indicate otherwise.

Cold Chemical Sterilization

The most common form of cold chemical sterilization used in the OR is peracetic acid (Steris system). This method of sterilization provides chemical irrigation of the item for 30 to 45 minutes at temperatures of 122°F to 133°F. This method can be used only for items that can be fully immersed in fluid (e.g., some cameras, scopes and cords).

Manufacturer's instructions for use of the Steris system must be followed to ensure that the items are properly sterilized. All items must be cleaned and all visible soil removed before being placed in the Steris pan. A special chemical indicator must be placed inside the pan with every load that is run. When the load is finished its cycle, the indicator must be checked before the items are placed on the sterile field. The items must be used immediately after processing and should not be stored for later use as sterility cannot be ensured with storage.

Caution: When handling the cup that must be placed in the Steris machine (see Fig. 1-22) before it is used, remember that the cup contains 35% peracetic acid, which can cause severe burns and blindness if it comes in contact with unprotected skin or eyes. Personal protective attire such as eyewear, gloves

FIGURE 1-22 Steris machine.

FIGURE 1–23 Cidex soaking tub.

and long sleeves (gown or jacket) should be worn when removing the cup from the package and placing it into the machine. The same attire should be worn when removing the used cup from the machine at the end of the cycle.

Another cold chemical that can be used to sterilize immersible items is glutaraldehyde (Cidex or Cidex OPA). The problem with using glutaraldehyde as a sterilant is that, in order for something to be deemed sterile, it must be soaked for about 10 hours in a tub of solution (see Fig. 1-23). This long soaking time makes it impractical to use in most cases in the OR. It is, however, used as a high-level disinfectant for endoscopes. *Caution:* Before placing any scope to soak in the solution, make sure it is *clean* and *dry*. Any bioburden or water left on the item can negatively affect the concentration of the solution, rendering it less effective.

Gas Plasma Sterilization

Gas plasma sterilization is a relatively new method of sterilization that employs the use of low-temperature hydrogen peroxide gas plasma technology. Items that are heat or moisture sensitive can be safely sterilized using this method.

This technology came about as an alternative to ethylene oxide (EO) sterilization, which is discussed in the following section. The by-products of gas plasma sterilization are oxygen and water, making it safer to use than EO sterilization. There is no exposure to hazardous materials. This system does not require aeration or ventilation procedures; therefore, the cycle time is shorter than with EO (1 hour for gas plasma versus up to 24 hours for EO). The system does have some limitations; linens, liquids and cellulose cannot be sterilized using this system. With some of the Sterrad systems there may be limits on the length and diameter of lumened instruments that can be effectively sterilized. *Always* refer to manufacturer's instructions before sterilizing any equipment or supplies.

Ethylene Oxide (Gas) Sterilization

EO is a flammable, toxic liquid that is combined with inert gas to produce sterilization. This type of sterilization is used for delicate items; that is, those that cannot withstand heat, pressure or moisture. EO penetrates wrappers and other materials that other sterilization methods may not. As with all sterilization methods, items must be thoroughly cleaned prior to sterilization.

The main disadvantage to EO is the toxicity. Any sterile processing center that uses EO must have devices throughout the area that monitor for leaks or unsafe levels of EO. If a leak is detected, the area must be evacuated and a hazardous materials team called in to deal with the problem. Exposure to EO has been associated with leukemia, respiratory damage, possible birth defects and neurological damage.

Items that have been sterilized with EO must be aerated to rid them of any residual gas. Aeration time varies item to item and be anywhere from 2 to 32 hours.

The long cycle time and the toxicity of the gas, as well as the expense of monitoring and maintaining the system, are causing some institutions to stop using EO sterilization completely and replace it with gas plasma systems.

Radiation Sterilization

The use of ionized radiation to sterilize equipment and supplies is extremely expensive and is used in the setting of medical device manufacturing plants.

This type of sterilization has strict guidelines and standards that must be adhered to in order to ensure the safety of personnel as well as the sterility of items.

OPERATING ROOM ATTIRE

When you work in the OR you are asked to surrender your "street clothes" and wear special attire. The purpose of this attire is threefold:

1. To protect the patient and OR from contamination you could have brought in on your street clothes
2. To contain any of your body's shedding skin or hair
3. To protect you from contact with body fluids or soil

The basic OR attire consists of scrub suit (or in some instances a scrub dress), mask, hat or cap, eye protection and, in some instances, shoe covers. The circulator or other non-scrubbed personnel also may wear a cover jacket. Additional attire for scrubbed personnel includes sterile gown and sterile gloves.

Although institutional policies may vary, it is recommended that OR personnel wear only attire that has been hospital (or institutional) laundered, not laundered at home. Institutional laundering of scrub attire helps ensure that it has been subjected to consistent and specialized cleaning standards that aid in keeping bacterial counts low.

Before describing each of the components of scrub attire, I want to say a few words about the wearing of *jewelry* in the OR. Institutional policies may vary; however, it is a recommended practice that NO jewelry be worn in the OR. Jewelry has been found to harbor microorganisms making it a potential source of contamination. Earrings or necklaces that are not fully contained under the scrub attire could come loose and fall into the surgical field or the wound. Jewelry could become contaminated with blood or other particles and pose a risk to personnel wearing it or others who contact it.

Scrub Suit

Most scrub suits consist of a top and pair of pants (see Fig. 1-24), although some institutions also offer the option to wear scrub dresses. This attire is made of lint-free material that can stand up to the rigors of institutional laundering.

Scrub suits should be close fitting to keep the material from "blousing" out, which could contaminate the sterile field, but they should not be so tight that they produce chafing or are offensive to others. Tunic-style tops should be tucked into the pants to avoid potentially contaminating the field if they are allowed to hang loose. If the pants have drawstrings at the top, the strings should be tucked into the pants to avoid any potential contact with sterile items.

Scrub suits should be changed daily or whenever they become contaminated with blood or body fluids (including excess perspiration). Institutional policy also may dictate that they be changed following certain isolation cases (e.g., MRSA); be sure to know the policies of your OR.

Masks

Masks are worn to protect the operative area from the airborne contamination that everyone generates when they breathe, talk, cough or sneeze. Masks are worn whenever you enter a restricted area of the OR suite, when you are near a scrub sink where personnel are scrubbing in preparation for entering the sterile field, or when you are in an area where sterile instruments are processed and stored. Institutional policies vary about which areas of the OR suite are "restricted"; it is imperative to know the layout and policies of your OR.

An additional function of a surgical mask is to protect the wearer from any spraying blood, body fluids and pieces of matter during the surgical procedure. The mask must be worn properly in order to do its job correctly; namely, block droplets and filter the air. The mask should cover *both* the mouth and nose because both are potential sources of airborne contamination. It should fit snugly; mold the pliable insert over the bridge of the nose to ensure a good fit. The ties should be tied at the top of the head and around the back of the neck to prevent unfiltered breath from escaping out the sides. The mask should be either on or taken off and discarded; it should not be worn dangling around the neck. Masks should be changed *after each case*. The mask should be removed by handling it by the strings, not the face part (this is the most contaminated part of the mask and therefore handling it should be avoided). Hands should be washed after removing the mask and disposing of it in the trash.

Masks come in several styles (see Fig. 1-25), including those that have a built-in face shield to protect the eyes from splash.

Laser Masks

There are special masks that need to be worn during procedures that involve the use of lasers (see Fig. 1-26). These masks are designed to filter out smaller particles than regular surgical masks (particle filtration of 0.1 μm). Laser use produces smaller particles when it destroys tissue cells, thus necessitating the use of a higher filtration mask to protect the wearer from possibly inhaling these smaller particles. Some institutions recommend or require the use of laser mask for specific procedures (e.g., electrosurgical removal of condylomata).

Hats and Caps

A hat or cap that covers *all* hair (including facial hair) must be worn in the restricted and semi-restricted areas of the OR. The purpose of the hat is to reduce contamination from hair or dander. There are several styles of cap or hat (see Fig. 1-27) that can be worn, but the important thing is that it completely covers all hair.

OR hats are made of disposable, lint-free material. They should be changed daily or when they become grossly contaminated or wet. Some institutions allow the wearing of individual cloth hats or caps in the OR, whereas others do not. This is an institutional decision; you need to check the policies of your OR before assuming it is acceptable to wear a cloth cap or hat. Cloth caps should be placed in the hospital laundry at the end of the day (or if grossly contaminated) to be cleaned; a cap that

FIGURE 1-24 OR personnel wearing scrub attire—shirt and drawstrings tucked inside the pants; cap on.

FIGURE 1–25 A) Fluid shield mask. B) Regular mask.

FIGURE 1–27 A) Cap. B) Hat.

FIGURE 1–26 Laser mask.

is worn for multiple days without being laundered is a source of contamination.

Recommended practices state that the cap or hat should be put on before donning your scrub suit to help prevent shedding of hair and dander onto clean scrub attire.

Eye Protection: Which personnel have to wear eye protection varies by institutional policy. Some institutions require *everyone* in the OR to wear eye protection while a procedure is being performed, whereas others may require only scrubbed personnel to wear eye protection and non-scrubbed personnel to don it when there is a chance they could contact blood, body fluid or tissue. Make sure to check your institution's policy regarding the wearing of eye protection.

Eye protection (see Fig. 1-28) must cover the eyes from the top of the eyebrows to the top of the surgical mask while protecting the sides of the face along the temples (this protects

FIGURE 1-28 Eyewear (disposable and non-disposable types).

the eyes from splash or tissue coming in around the sides). Regular eyeglasses DO NOT meet standards for eye protection because they do not provide protection along the sides of the eyes. In order to make eyeglasses meet the requirements, eye shields made for this purpose can be purchased and attached to them. Goggles and surgical masks with faceshields are other acceptable types of eye protection. The type of eye protection that one wears depends on personal preference, comfort, ability to see to perform duties, availability and cost.

Cover Jacket: Non-scrubbed personnel may choose to wear a cover jacket or "scrub jacket" (see Fig. 1-29). These jackets

FIGURE 1-29 Scrub jacket.

provide some warmth as well as helping to contain shed skin, thus decreasing contamination in the OR. If these jackets are to be worn, it is recommended that they be close fitting and that the front be buttoned or snapped closed. Jackets that are very loose or are "flapping" open in the front may pose a contamination risk by brushing up against sterile items. Jackets should be made of material that does not shed (e.g., in most places, fleece jackets are not acceptable because they shed fibers, thus increasing contamination). Wearing of these jackets is governed by institutional policy; be sure you know what your policy says before you assume it is acceptable to wear one.

Shoe Covers: The wearing of shoe covers varies by institutional policy. Even if your institution does not require the wearing of shoe covers, you may want to consider doing so, especially in cases where there is a high likelihood of your shoes becoming wet (e.g., arthroscopy or cesarean section). This helps to protect your shoes, socks and feet from becoming contaminated with water, blood and body fluids. If you wear shoe covers, they need to be changed daily or when they become soiled, torn or wet. They must be removed when you are leaving the OR area.

Shoe covers are available in two lengths (see Fig. 1-30). One length comes up to the ankle and covers the foot and shoe. This length is worn for most cases. The second length extends up the leg to the knees. This longer length is worn during arthroscopies or other surgeries where there is a potential for a large amount of water and body fluid to make its way onto the floor.

Nonsterile Gloves: Although not necessarily considered part of OR "attire," nonsterile gloves are an important part of personal protective attire. These gloves are worn by nonsterile personnel whenever there is any chance of contact with blood, body fluids or tissues (e.g., handling specimens or specimen containers, performing intubation, handling soiled linen or instruments). Gloves must be worn by all personnel when cleaning the room between cases. After use, gloves are discarded in the trash (being careful not to touch the contaminated part with your bare skin) and then hands need to be washed. Gloves are not impervious to all contaminants; therefore, wearing gloves does not mean that your hands are clean after you remove the gloves. *Wearing gloves is NOT a substitute for handwashing!*

Nonsterile gloves are available in sizes small, medium, large and extra large (see Fig. 1-31). They are made from latex and nonlatex materials. Many institutions have switched to nonlatex gloves to lessen health care workers' exposure to latex.

X-Ray Gowns (Lead): Another piece of "attire" that OR personnel are required to wear during certain procedures is a lead apron (also referred to as a *lead gown*). The apron should have an attached thyroid shield. If the thyroid shield is not attached to the gown, then a separate thyroid shield should be used. The lead apron and thyroid shield are put on over the scrubs but

FIGURE 1–30 A) Short shoe cover. B) Long shoe cover.

FIGURE 1–31 Nonsterile gloves.

underneath the sterile gown of scrubbed personnel, and they are put on over the scrubs of nonsterile personnel.

The lead apron is used whenever there is going to be exposure to radiation (i.e., x-rays or fluoroscopy) during the procedure. There are several styles of lead aprons: one and two piece (vest and skirt), ones that completely wrap around the body and ones that cover only the person's front and sides. Which style you choose depends on the procedure being done and the type of x-ray machinery being used. For example, lead aprons that are used when the mini C-arm is being used have a thinner lead lining because exposure to radiation is minimal. These aprons cannot be used when other types of

x-ray machinery are in use because they do not offer enough protection.

Whenever possible, lead shields or aprons and thyroid shields are placed on the patient to protect the reproductive organs and thyroid from radiation exposure.

Sterile Attire

Sterile attire is worn by scrubbed personnel during the surgical procedure. Sterile attire consists of sterile gown and gloves. Some institutions may require that sterile hoods be worn during joint replacement surgery.

Sterile Gown: The sterile gown is designed to cover the body of the scrubbed person from the base of the neck to below the knees. This provides a sterile barrier between the person's unsterile scrub attire and the sterile field.

The gown is only sterile if the integrity of the package is not compromised. If the package has a hole, is torn, is wet or the package seal is compromised, the gown is no longer sterile and must be discarded.

Once donned, the only parts of the gown that are considered sterile are (1) the front of the gown from the waist up to mid-chest level, and (2) the sleeves up to 2 inches above the elbow. The stockinette sleeve cuffs are NOT considered sterile as they are not impervious; therefore, the sleeve cuffs must be completely covered by the cuff of the sterile gloves at all times. The reason that only these limited areas are considered sterile is because they are the only parts of the gown that the scrubbed person can see and therefore ensure that they have not been inadvertently contaminated.

Sterile gowns are available in cloth or paper (see Fig. 1-33). Which type of gown a person uses is based on personal preference and availability. Most gowns are available in sizes large and extra large, and some styles are available in sizes up to triple-extra large.

Sterile Gloves: Sterile gloves have been specially processed to render them microbe-free. They come in sealed packages, the inside of which is considered sterile (except for a 1-inch

Care of Lead Aprons

■ Prior to use, lead aprons should be checked to make sure they are not cracked or torn. Cracks or tears can compromise the integrity of the shield and decrease its effectiveness.

■ Lead aprons should be hung up on appropriate hangers when not in use; they should not be folded or heaped in piles (see Fig. 1-32).

■ Lead aprons should be x-rayed at least yearly to check for breaks in the integrity of the lead.

FIGURE 1–32 A) Proper way to hang lead aprons. B) Improper way to hang lead aprons.

margin around the edges). Sterile gloves can be made of latex or nonlatex material (see Fig. 1-34). They come sized in half sizes, generally ranging from size 5½ to 9. Most sterile gloves are now powder-free, but special care must be taken if your institution is still using powdered gloves.

It is generally recommended that scrubbed personnel *double glove;* that is, *put on a colored underglove and top it with an outer glove. Double gloving provides many advantages:*

■ In the event of a needlestick, the health care provider is exposed to less contamination from the needle. It has been shown that fewer microbes are left on the needle point after puncturing through two layers; microbes are wiped off as the needle passes through each layer.

FIGURE 1–33 Paper and cloth gowns.

Powdered Gloves

■ Gloves that contain powder have the potential to cause adhesions at the surgical site. Powdered sterile gloves should be rinsed in sterile saline or wiped with a sterile saline-soaked sponge before beginning surgery.

■ Discard the sponge used to wipe the gloves into the kick bucket or other proper sponge receptacle.

FIGURE 1–34 A) Latex glove package. B) Nonlatex glove package.

■ In the event that the scrubbed person touches a contaminated instrument, tray or the patient's unprepped skin, only the outer glove(s) need to be changed. The scrub person can change the outer glove(s) him- or herself without waiting for assistance.

■ Wearing a pair of colored undergloves has been shown to make it easier to detect a hole in the outer gloves. The outer gloves can be changed immediately, thus decreasing chances of contamination by a hole going unnoticed.

■ If the outer gloves become torn or have a hole, there is still a protective barrier between the patient and the scrub person. The patient is not accidently exposed to microbes from the scrub person's skin and the scrub person is not exposed to blood or body fluid from the patient.

What size glove combination a person wears is a matter of personal preference and comfort. Each person should try different combination of glove sizes for both inner and outer gloves until a combination is found that allows for the performance of duties without restriction on the nerves or blood flow. *Hint:* If you get numb fingers, try an inner glove that is ½ to 1 size larger. If you still have problems, increase the outer glove size.

Gloves come in a variety of materials: heavier for "orthopedic" gloves, softer for those with sensitive skin, latex and non-latex material. The type of glove used depends on personal preference and patient and personnel allergy history. Whether or not you can use latex gloves and when they can be used is dependent on institutional policy. Some ORs are latex-free and latex gloves are not allowed at all. Make sure you know your institution's policy regarding the use of latex gloves.

Sterile Space Suit: The so-named sterile space suit consists of a regular sterile gown and a sterile hood that completely covers the head and face (see Fig. 1-35). The hood has a convex clear full-face shield and resembles a hood used by astronauts. The hood has a self-contained, battery-operated fan in the top to allow for ventilation. The fan is attached to a plastic headpiece that is placed on the scrub personnel's head prior to scrubbing. The battery pack is worn on the person's waistband. The sterile hood is placed on over the plastic frame when the person gowns and gloves.

This type of attire is required in some institutions during total joint replacement surgery. The theory behind this attire is that it cuts down on contamination from respiratory droplets and uncovered hair.

OPERATING ROOM TABLE

The OR table (also referred to as the *OR bed*) is the central focal point of the OR suite. It is the most important piece of furniture in the room; this is where the patient is placed and the procedure takes place. The table is located near the center of the room so that there is enough room to move equipment, instrument tables and personnel around the patient on both sides and at the bottom. The head of the bed is reserved for anesthesia personnel, supplies and machinery.

Operating tables come in a variety of styles. Older tables are operated manually, using cranks to position the patient, but all newer tables are electrical and are operated using remote controls (see Fig. 1-36).

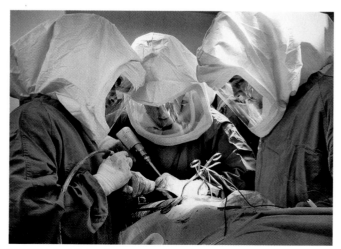

FIGURE 1–35 Sterile space suit hood. © imageofsurgery.com)

As with any piece of medical equipment, it is important to know how to use the OR table in the room you are assigned (see Fig. 1-37). Make sure you know the manufacturer's instructions for table use. All personnel should receive instruction on the tables being used in their institution as part of their orientation as well as when any new table is purchased. Failure to be familiar with proper table use could result in surgery delays, increased anesthesia time for the patient (while personnel try to

FIGURE 1-36 A) Manual OR table. B) Electric OR table.

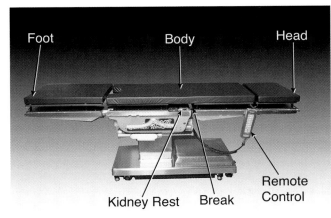

FIGURE 1-37 OR table parts.

> **WATCH OUT!** **Operating Room Table Weight Limits**
>
> ■ Some older manual models of OR tables have a 350-lb weight limit.
>
> ■ Some older electric models of OR tables have a 500- to 550-lb weight limit.
>
> ■ Some newer models of OR tables have capacities of 1000 lbs plus, but only in certain positions (e.g., supine); the weight limit is lower if the patient is in lithotomy or other position.
>
> It is imperative that you know the weight limit of the OR table you are using PRIOR to placing the patient on it. Failure to use the proper table for large patients could result in severe injury to the patient or staff.

figure out how to work the bed during a procedure) or injury to the patient or staff.

Parts of an Operating Room Table

Headpiece: The headpiece is a removable padded section attached at the head of the bed (usually with metal rods or bars). This section can be adjusted up or down to aid in airway maintenance. The headpiece can be removed to allow for attachment of other headrests such as a Mayfield headrest (neurosurgery) or a horseshoe headrest. The headpiece also can be removed and placed at the bottom of the table for some gynecological procedures.

Body: The body of the table usually consists of two padded pieces with a "break" in between them. The break allows for each piece to be flexed or extended independently for patient positioning (e.g., Fowler's or sitting position). There is a metal bar in the break area that can be moved up and down. This bar is known as a *kidney rest* and is used to elevate the flank area for better exposure during renal procedures.

Footpiece: The footpiece or bottom of the bed is a padded removable section where the patient's lower legs and feet rest. The footpiece can be flexed or extended independently of the rest of the bed for patient positioning, or it can be moved out of the way during vaginal procedures.

Operating Table Attachments

Mayfield Headrest: This attachment (see Fig. 1-38) is used for some craniotomy procedures. The Mayfield headrest generally is used to hold the head still when the patient is prone or in Fowler's (sitting) position. The headrest is attached to the patient's skull using sterile pins. This headrest is attached to the patient by the *surgeon* and positioning is done with the surgeon present.

Gardner Tongs: Gardner tongs (see Fig. 1-39) are used to apply cervical traction to patients with cervical spine fractures. They are attached into each side of the patient's skull using sterile pins. Weight is attached to a rope loop that goes over a pulley to create the traction.

FIGURE 1-38 Mayfield headrest.

FIGURE 1-40 Horseshoe headrest.

FIGURE 1-39 Gardner tongs.

FIGURE 1-41 Arm board.

Horseshoe Headrest: As its name implies, the horseshoe headrest is shaped like a horseshoe (see Fig. 1-40). This headrest can be used to support the patient's forehead when he or she is in the prone position or the back of the head when he or she is supine. It is attached to the OR bed where the headpiece would normally be attached.

Arm Boards: Arm boards are attached to each side of the bed to support the patient's outstretched arms (see Fig. 1-41). The boards are padded, but extra padding may be needed in the areas of the shoulder, elbow, wrist or hand, depending on the patient. Although some arm boards are interchangeable (fit more than one OR table), some are not; make sure you

have the proper arm boards before positioning the patient on the table.

Shoulder Braces: Padded shoulder braces are attached to the head of the bed when the patient is placed in the Trendelenburg position (see Fig. 1-42). They are used to prevent the patient from sliding upward, off the top of the bed. Care should be taken when using these braces as improper positioning of the braces could cause undo pressure to the nerves and muscles of the shoulder, resulting in injury to the patient. Shoulder braces should be applied only by personnel familiar with their use.

Toboggan: Also known as a *sled* or *arm shield,* the toboggan is a Plexiglas three quarter box-shaped device used to brace the arm or leg at the patient's side, preventing the appendage from falling off the table (see Fig. 1-43). The device is held in place by sliding it under the mattress.

Allen Arm Support: The Allen arm support (see Fig. 1-44) can be used to hold the hand and wrist in the prone, lateral or seated position. The handrest is malleable to allow for

WATCH OUT! **Hyperextension of the Arms**

A patient's arm should NEVER be extended >90 degrees on an arm board. Extending a patient's arm >90 degrees could result in damage to the brachial plexis with resulting temporary or permanent nerve damage.

FIGURE 1–42 Shoulder braces.

FIGURE 1–43 Toboggan.

flexibility in positioning. The arm rest is made of metal; therefore, padding (e.g., gel pad) must be applied before placing the patient's hand and wrist on it.

Hand Table: The hand table (see Fig. 1-45) is a rectangular or hourglass-shaped folding table used to support the entire arm and hand during surgery. It attaches to the side of the OR table and can be moved easily for repositioning. It has one or two telescoping legs to support the distal end of the table. It is available in several sizes ranging from 14 to 23 inches in width to 29 to 38 inches in length.

Beach Chair: Also known as a *captain's chair,* the beach chair is an attachment used to support the patient in an upright sitting position for shoulder surgery. The patient's head is strapped into a headrest and the nonoperative arm is strapped to the patient's waist. Specially designed disposable padding is used with this device (see Fig. 1-46).

Footboard: The footboard (see Fig. 1-47) is a rectangular metal board that attaches to the bottom of OR table at a right

FIGURE 1–44 A) Allen arm support. B) Allen arm support with gel pad.

angle. The footboard is used to prevent the patient who is in reverse Trendelenburg position from sliding off the bottom of the table. Place padding on the footboard to prevent pressure

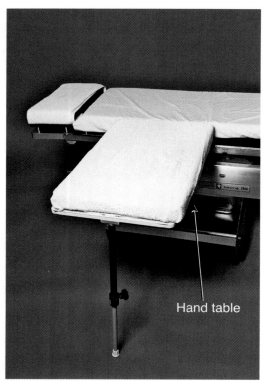

FIGURE 1–45 Hand table.

injury to the patient's feet. This attachment can also be used as a "shelf" during vaginal procedures by attaching it at a right angle to the footpiece of the bed that is lowered all the way down.

Stirrups

Candy Cane Stirrups: Also known as *sling stirrups*, candy cane stirrups (see Fig. 1-48) support the foot and heel of the patient in lithotomy position. These stirrups are used for gynecological

---

WATCH OUT! | **Placing the Patient's Legs in Stirrups**

- When placing the patient in stirrups, both legs must be lifted *slowly, at the same time,* by two people. Failure to do this could result in injury to the spine or hips.

- Removing the patient from stirrups requires two people to lower the legs *slowly, at the same time,* to prevent stress on the patient's lower back.

- If legs are lowered too quickly, hypotension could occur.

- Caution needs to be taken to make sure the hip flexion is not too severe as this can damage the femoral nerves.

- Patients with knee or hip replacements or those with limited range of motion should be positioned while awake in order to avoid damage/severe pain due to hyperextension of the knee or hip joints

---

FIGURE 1–46 A) Beach chair. B) Padding for beach chair.

FIGURE 1-47 Footboard.

FIGURE 1-48 Candy cane stirrups.

FIGURE 1-49 Knee-crutch stirrups.

procedures. Care must be taken to make sure the side of the patient's lower leg is NOT resting on the metal post of the candy cane stirrup. Do not place the sling directly over the Achilles area as pressure could cause injury to the peroneal nerve.

Knee-Crutch Stirrups: These stirrups provide support under the knee and areas just above and below the knee (see Fig. 1-49). They are generally used for short-duration knee arthroscopy or cystoscopy procedures. Care must be taken to

properly pad and position the stirrups to prevent popliteal nerve damage.

Boot Stirrups: Rapidly becoming the stirrup of choice for many gynecological and rectal procedures, the boot stirrup provides support to the patient's foot and entire lower leg (see Fig. 1-50). This type of stirrup is completely adjustable both vertically and for abduction. The boot is padded, but care must be taken to properly place the patient's leg in the boot (make sure the heel is all the way back into the boot) to prevent nerve injury. There are several manufacturers of boot-type stirrups so make sure you are familiar with the operation of the stirrups (how to raise, lower and abduct them) used at your facility.

Frames for Lumbar Surgery

Wilson Frame: The Wilson frame (see Fig. 1-51) is used to support a patient's torso in a flexed, prone position. This frame is used for surgeries of the lumbar spine including laminectomy, diskectomy and microdiskectomy as well as insertion of bladder control stimulators. It consists of two padded half circles mounted on a frame that is placed under the prone patient's torso. Using a crank system, the supports can be raised or lowered to achieve the desired amount of flexion. The supports also can be adjusted laterally to fit multiple patient body types.

FIGURE 1–50 Boot stirrups.

FIGURE 1–52 Andrews frame.

FIGURE 1–51 Wilson frame.

Miscellaneous Tables

Orthopedic (Fracture) Bed: The orthopedic or fracture table (see Fig. 1-54) is used for procedures such as hip nailing, femoral rodding, tibial nailing and hip arthroscopy. The table has leg positioners that can be moved laterally to move the nonoperative leg out of the way and allow for C-arm access. Traction and rotation can be applied to either leg. There are multiple accessories that can be used with this table to allow it to be configured for many types of procedures.

Top Sliding Table: The tabletop slides up to the head or down to the foot allowing for imaging access to any part of the body (see Fig. 1-55). These tables can be used for any surgical procedure in which C-arm or other imaging is expected to be needed such as some urology, major endovascular, orthopedic or general surgery. Like other OR tables, they can be rotated or flexed as needed.

Andrews Frame: The Andrews frame (see Fig. 1-52) is used to support the patient in knee-chest position for surgery on the lumbar spine. This frame is mounted on the bottom end of an OR table where the footpiece has been removed. The patient is anesthetized in a supine position and carefully rolled prone and into knee-chest position on the frame. Ventilation is a major concern with the use of this frame— make sure the chest has room to expand once the patient is positioned.

Jackson Table: The Jackson table (see Fig. 1-53) is a frame with interchangeable accessories that allow it to be adapted for cervical, thoracic and lumbar surgical procedures. There is a flat surface for positioning the patient for cervical spine surgery, and a Wilson frame that can be mounted on the Jackson table for lumbar surgery along with a sling footpiece or flat footpiece. There is a top that can be placed over the patient and secured to allow for "flipping" the patient 180 degrees.

WATCH OUT! | **Orthopedic Table**

- The orthopedic table can be configured in several ways. Make sure you know which configuration is needed for the procedure being performed.

- Make sure you know how to use the table and accessories BEFORE the procedure. If you are unsure, ask someone experienced with its use and consult the user manual.

- Make sure that the perineal post is well padded. The patient's perineal area should NOT rest directly against the post.

- Traction to the affected leg should be directed/applied by the *surgeon*. Make sure the foot is secure in the boot before applying the traction. Failure to do so could result in the foot slipping out, causing further damage from the fracture or damage to the skin of the foot.

FIGURE 1–53 Three configurations for the Jackson table. A) With Wilson frame. B) With flat frame. C) With padded bolsters.

OPERATING ROOM FURNITURE

One of the first things that new personnel in an OR environment notice is that the furniture is different from any other patient care area. The OR furniture is generally made of stainless steel (for ease of cleaning), has wheels to make it portable and is designed to perform a specific purpose. It is not decorative but plain and utilitarian. In this section, the most common pieces of furniture (except for the beds, which have their own section) are described.

All OR furniture should be wiped down thoroughly (all surfaces) with a hospital-grade disinfectant at the beginning of the day and between cases according to your institutional policy.

Back Table: The back table (also known as an *instrument table*) is a large one- or a two-tiered stainless steel table that, when covered with a sterile drape, is used to hold the sterile instruments and supplies (see Fig. 1-56). The sterile pack is opened on the back table (creating a sterile field), and then the instruments, sutures and other sterile supplies are opened onto it. If a large number of instruments or supplies are needed for the case, more than one back table may be used.

FIGURE 1–54 A) Fracture table closed. B) Fracture table opened.

FIGURE 1–55 Top-sliding table.

FIGURE 1–56 Back table.

Back tables come in a variety of sizes and heights. The table may have one or two top shelves. The model with two top shelves is generally used for vascular or orthopedic surgery, and both top shelves are covered with a sterile drape. Some back tables have a bottom shelf about 12 to 18 inches under the top shelf. On these models, the bottom shelf is not covered with a drape and NOT considered sterile.

Mayo Stand: The Mayo stand is covered with a special sterile drape made specifically for that purpose and is used to set up instruments that need to be readily available for the case (see Fig. 1-57). The instruments placed on the Mayo stand vary depending on the case but should be kept to a minimum to avoid disorganization and wasted time hunting for needed items. The space on top of the Mayo stand is limited; use it only for the items needed to start the case (e.g., scalpels and superficial retractors) and those that will be used repeatedly (e.g., common rings such as kochers, allis and hemostats; Mayo and Metzenbaum scissors; smooth and tissue forceps) on it. The rest of the instruments should be organized on the back table. Instruments can be removed and replaced with others (e.g., deeper retractors) as the surgery progresses.

Mayo stands come in a variety of styles. The height on most Mayo stands can be adjusted from 36 to 62 inches to allow them to be moved up to the field, over the patient. Height adjustment is made either by stepping on a foot button or pulling a hand lever, depending on the model. Standard Mayo stands have a tray surface area of 12 × 19 inches or 16 × 21 inches. Extra large Mayo stands (used mostly in orthopedic or neurosurgical procedures) have a surface area of 20 × 25 inches. The extra large stand requires an extra large sterile Mayo cover.

Utility Table: The utility table (also called a *prep table*) is a small stainless steel table (see Fig. 1-58) that can be used for a variety of things. When it is covered with a sterile drape, it can be used to hold the basins and other supplies used

FIGURE 1-57 A) Large Mayo stand. B) Draped large Mayo stand. C) Regular Mayo stand. D) Draped regular Mayo stand.

for the skin prep or as a separate small sterile field (e.g., for a local anesthesia supply set-up or for a sigmoidoscopy set-up). Unsterile, it can be used to hold paperwork, specimen containers, scales (for weighing specimens) or other items.

Utility tables come in a variety of styles, some with drawers and some without. They are small, with a surface area of about 16 × 20 inches.

Mobile Instrument Stand: The mobile instrument stand (see Fig. 1-59) is a small, single-post stand that can be covered with a sterile drape and used to hold instruments and supplies for a minor surgical or dental case. The surface area is 12 × 19 inches and the height is adjustable from 31 to 50 inches. Unlike a Mayo stand, the mobile instrument stand is made to go beside the OR bed, not over the patient's body or feet.

FIGURE 1–58 Utility table.

Kick Bucket: The kick bucket (see Fig. 1-60) is a stainless steel 13-quart bucket set into a round, rolling stainless steel frame. The bucket is commonly used to contain dirty sponges discarded from the field. The sponges are discarded into the bucket; the circulator (using proper standard precautions) may drape the sponges over the side of the bucket for ease of counting. Some institutions require that discarded sponges be placed in plastic impervious sponge count bags for counting, not draped on the side of the bucket. Check your institution's policies and procedures.

Ring Stand: The ring stand (also known as a *basin stand*) is a round stainless steel ring mounted on a rolling stand (see Fig. 1-61). The large (8.5 quart) sterile basin is opened in this stand with the wrapper opened outward to cover the top and side of the stand, creating a sterile field. The sterile basin can then be used as a place into which to organize drapes or gowns or to open other sterile items.

Ring stands are available as single or double (holds two basins side by side) models. They have open frames to allow easy access from any side and may or may not have a shelf underneath.

Standing Stool: The standing stool (also known as a *step stool*) comes in a variety of styles (see Fig. 1-62). Like the name implies, this stool is made for members of the surgical team to stand on during a procedure for better visualization of the surgical field. The important thing to check on a standing

FIGURE 1–59 Mobile instrument stand.

FIGURE 1–60 Kick bucket.

FIGURE 1–61 Ring stand.

FIGURE 1–63 Sitting stool.

FIGURE 1–62 Step stool.

can be individually adjusted in height and also radially (outward or inward). The height of the stool can be adjusted from 19 to 28 inches using a foot control.

Surgical Spotlights: Surgical spotlights come in a variety of sizes and configurations, but they are made for one purpose: to provide a concentrated beam of light into the surgical field that allows for better visualization (see Fig. 1-65). The focus of the beam and beam location are controlled by sterile light handles that are inserted into the lights before making the first incision.

stool is that all four rubber feet on the stool are solid and intact; otherwise, the stool may be wobbly and can pose a safety hazard.

Standing stools are 11¼ inches high and come in regular (350 lb weight limit) or bariatric (600 lb weight limit) styles.

Sitting Stool: Sitting stools are used during surgical procedures when it is more advantageous for the surgeon and staff to sit during the procedure rather than stand (e.g., hand surgeries, vaginal procedures). These stools adjust in height from 17 to 24 inches (see Fig. 1-63). Depending on the model, they are adjusted by turning the seat, which is mounted on a large screw-type pole or using a pneumatic lever. The seats are padded for comfort. Be sure to check the weight capacity of the stools in your institution before use as some have weight capacities as low as 250 lb.

Specialty Surgery Stool: Commonly used for ophthalmologic; ear, nose and throat or microsurgery, the specialty surgery stool is more like a chair (see Fig. 1-64). It has two armrests to support and help steady the surgeon's forearms. The armrests

FIGURE 1–64 Specialty surgery stool.

FIGURE 1–65 Surgical spotlights.

FIGURE 1–66 IV pole.

Most ORs have two or three surgical spotlights located above the surgical bed. The lights are mounted on arms so they can be moved and adjusted.

Surgical spotlights should be turned on and checked—at the beginning of the day and between cases—for burned out bulbs. Any bulbs that are burned out or dim should be changed before the start of the case to allow for maximum visualization of the surgical field. Spotlights should be wiped down with disinfectant at the beginning of the day and between cases according to your institution's infection control policies.

Intravenous Pole: Intravenous (IV) poles come in a variety of styles, but they are all used to hang IV fluid, medication or blood transfusion bags. The IV poles are mounted on a stand with wheels to allow for portability (see Fig. 1-66). They generally have two or four rings at the top for hanging the solution bags. The height is adjustable; generally, pediatric IV poles adjust from 56 to 89 inches and adult models adjust from 68 to 99 inches or 75 to 101 inches. Some IV poles come with a shelf to allow for pumps to be mounted onto them.

Irrigation Tower: An irrigation tower performs a function similar to an IV pole: it is made to hold bags of fluid. The differences between the irrigation tower and an IV pole are that the height of each arm (the metal hook that holds the bag) of the irrigation tower can be adjusted separately and that the irrigation tower is made to be stable even when it is holding large amounts of fluids (see Fig. 1-67). These towers are used when large amounts of irrigation fluid are expected to be used, such as during arthroscopic or cystoscopic procedures. The total capacity for fluid that can be hung on each tower varies by manufacturer; make sure you are familiar with the specific tower in your OR before use.

In-Line Gas and Electric Columns: ORs sometimes have the gas (e.g., nitrogen, oxygen and nitrous oxide), suction and electrical

FIGURE 1–67 Irrigation tower.

outlets built into columns, which vary in style and size, that are mounted on the ceiling (see Fig. 1-68). The advantage to the columns is that everything is housed in one area off the floor, lessening the number of cords running along the floor and thus decreasing potential tripping hazards.

X-Ray Viewing Box: Most ORs have one or more x-ray viewing boxes mounted on the wall (see Fig. 1-69). These illuminated boxes allow patient films to be viewed during the procedure. The most common configurations are single panel (14 × 17 inches) or double panel (28 × 17 inches). The boxes should be checked prior to the start of the case to ensure that they are functioning properly.

Picture Archiving and Communication System: The Picture Archiving and Communication System (PACS) allows institutions to archive a patient's radiological studies and retrieve them on a computer system installed in a remote location (e.g., the OR or an off-site location) (see Fig. 1-70). This system archives and retrieves not only regular x-ray films but also ultrasounds, magnetic resonance imaging scans, computed tomography scans, positron emission tomography scans, mammography and arteriography.

X-Ray Cassette Holder: There are many styles of x-ray cassette holders (see Fig. 1-71), but the ones used in ORs are small and mounted on wheels so that they can be moved easily. The height of the bars can be adjusted to accommodate several

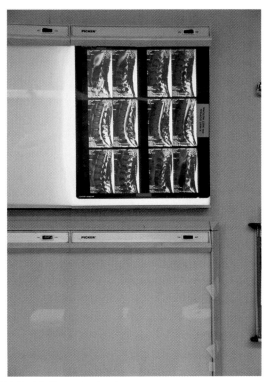

FIGURE 1-69 X-ray viewing box.

FIGURE 1-68 In-line column.

FIGURE 1-70 PACS system.

FIGURE 1–71 Cassette holder.

FIGURE 1–72 Lead door.

cassette sizes. These holders are used to hold the cassette in place when lateral x-rays are needed intraoperatively. The holders and cassette are not sterile; therefore, they must be draped (e.g., by using a sterile half drape) if they are to be moved close to the surgical field.

Lead Door: The lead door (also known as a *mobile barrier*) is used to shield staff from radiation during the taking of intraoperative x-rays. This type of door is mounted on wheels to allow for portability, and it is rolled to a location away from the sterile field. Staff stand behind it while taking x-rays. The door has clear lead windows (see Fig. 1-72) to allow staff to see the patient. Doors are available with 0.5 mm, 1.0 mm or 1.5 mm of lead protection.

ELECTROSURGICAL UNITS

The invention of electrosurgery helped to revolutionize the speed at which surgery was performed. Surgeons could now cut and cauterize tissue with the push of a button or a touch of the foot pedal instead of having to tie off each bleeding blood vessel individually. In today's modern surgical suite, some form of electrosurgery is used in most procedures. In this section, common types of electrosurgery (i.e., monopolar, bipolar and argon beam) as well parts of the electrosurgical unit (e.g., active and inactive electrodes, bipolar devices, argon beam wand and tips) are covered. Following this section are pages discussing electrosurgery

safety, what to do if the patient sustains a burn and simple troubleshooting.

Control Panel for the Electrosurgical Generator

There are several different models of electrosurgery generators available. Figure 1-73 shows one common type with the plugs and controls labeled. This figure is intended as a guide to basic features of most generators; refer to the instruction manual for specific information regarding the generators used in your institution.

FIGURE 1–73 Control panel of ESU.

Most electrosurgical units (ESU; also referred to as *ESU generator*) are capable of producing two modes of current: monopolar and bipolar.

Monopolar Electrosurgery

Monopolar is the most commonly used form of electrosurgical current for many surgeries. In the monopolar mode, electrical current goes from the ESU generator to the handpiece (called the *pencil;* this is the *active electrode*), where it contacts the tissue. Once the tissue is cut or cauterized, the current travels through the patient's body until it gets to the grounding pad (called the *dispersive pad;* this is the *inactive electrode).* The current exits through the grounding pad back to the generator and ground.

When using the monopolar current mode, it is essential that the patient have a properly placed grounding or dispersive pad (*inactive* or *passive electrode*) on their skin (see Fig. 1-74). Most modern ESU generators will not work unless the grounding pad is plugged into the proper outlet. Many ESU generators will also sound an alarm (and not work) if the pad has come loose or is folded on itself. However, the staff person applying the dispersive pad is responsible to make sure it is *properly* applied. An improperly or misplaced pad has the potential to cause burns to the patient's skin!

Monopolar Handpieces and Tips

The *active electrode* is what the surgeon uses to cut or cauterize tissue. The most common form of active electrode is the pencil (see Figs. 1-75 and 1-76). A tip is inserted into the pencil. The type of tip depends on what surgery is being performed.

Styles of Tips

Common tips (see Fig. 1-77) for open procedures include spatula (flat blade), needle point (for working in small or delicate areas), ball tip or loop (for resection in such procedures as a loop electrosurgical excision procedure [LEEP]). Long extension tips are available (most commonly spatula and needle point) for working on tissue deep within a body cavity. Teflon-coated tips may be used when a great deal of cautery

Guidelines for Properly Placing a Dispersive (Grounding) Pad

- Prior to placement, inspect the pad for any tears, kinks in the cord, splits in the cord or other damage. Remove the plastic protective backing and check the gel to ensure that it is sticky and fresh, not dried out. DO NOT use a damaged pad; if there is any doubt about the integrity of the pad, toss it out and get a new one!
- Make sure the site is clean and dry. Remove any lotions or creams as necessary.
- DO NOT apply on excessively hairy areas. If necessary, shave the area prior to pad application.
- Place over a large muscle mass with good vascularization. Upper thigh and outer thigh are two of the best areas.
- Uniform, smooth skin contact is essential. The pad should not be folded, bunched up or torn. Pad should be placed AFTER final positioning of the patient to avoid damaging the pad or having the pad pull away from the skin.
- DO NOT apply over a bony prominence or over an area containing an artificial prosthesis (e.g., a total hip prosthesis). Excessive scar tissue at the site of the prosthesis can impede conduction.
- Apply the pad as close to the operative site as possible (e.g., for a patient undergoing an appendectomy, place the pad on the right thigh if possible).

FIGURE 1–75 Pencil electrode.

FIGURE 1–74 Grounding pad.

FIGURE 1–76 Suction electrode.

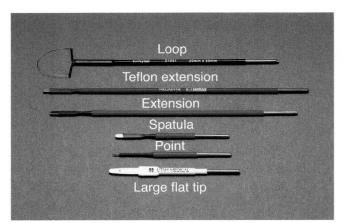

FIGURE 1-77 Loop, Teflon extension, extension tip, spatula, point, large flat tip.

FIGURE 1-78 Bipolar cord.

FIGURE 1-79 Bipolar forceps.

FIGURE 1-80 Argon beam machine.

is anticipated (these tips are easier to keep free of tissue debris). Endoscopic procedures require special electrodes that are long and thin. There are a variety of endoscopic electrodes including probes and graspers.

The pencil can be activated by pressing a button or stepping on the foot pedal. While the electrode is activated, the ESU makes an audible signal that alerts personnel that the tip is hot and therefore a potential hazard. These signals are intended for patient safety device and should never be disabled or turned down so low as to make them inaudible to personnel in the room.

Bipolar Electrosurgery

In bipolar electrosurgery, the current passes from one tine of the forceps to the other; the current never passes through the patient. The power is lower than what can be achieved with monopolar cautery and is used for cauterization during neurosurgery or on delicate tissue. The current does not pass through the patient, thus a dispersive (or grounding) pad is *not* needed.

Note: If the surgeon is going to be using *both* monopolar and bipolar current during the procedure, a dispersive electrode pad *must* be placed on the patient.

Special forceps are used to deliver bipolar current. The forceps are available in a wide variety of styles and plug into the ESU using a bipolar cord (see Fig. 1-78). Many of the forceps resemble regular grasping forceps (see Fig. 1-79) but with one important difference; these forceps have a plug on the end of the handle to plug them into the bipolar cord.

Argon Beam Coagulation

Argon beam coagulation (also referred to as *ABC* or *argon plasma coagulation*) uses a combination of argon gas and monopolar electrosurgery to coagulate tissue. Within the machine (see Fig. 1-80) the gas is ionized, making it electrically conductive. This provides a more efficient pathway for the current to travel along to the tissue. The tip of the instrument does not need to touch the tissue; the beam of ionized gas coagulates bleeders within 2 to 10 mm of the tip. Argon beam coagulation produces less tissue damage, less smoke plume and less charring than traditional electrosurgery methods.

A special instrument or wand (see Fig. 1-81) is needed when using the argon beam coagulation mode of the machine. On some argon beam machines, you can turn the gas tank off and use it with a traditional pencil as a monopolar device or

FIGURE 1-81 Argon beam wand.

plug it in for use with bipolar coagulation. Be sure to refer to the manufacturer's instruction book to see if the unit in your institution can be used this way.

Remember: Argon beam coagulation allows the beam to travel through the patient's body; therefore, a dispersive electrode (grounding pad) *must* be used.

Electrosurgical Safety

As with any electrical device, there are certain safety measures that should be followed when an ESU is in use:

- Know your machine. Only personnel knowledgeable about electrosurgical use and safety precautions should use the device. If you have questions, refer to the manufacturer's instructions.
- Check the unit for frayed cords or damaged plugs prior to use. If the electric cord is split, frayed or otherwise compromised or the prongs on the plug are bent, damaged or missing DO NOT use the machine. A different machine should be obtained and the damaged one checked by biomedical engineering.
- Do not store liquids on top of the machine. Spills could occur and cause electrical shock or shortage.
- Make sure the electrosurgical grounding pad (inactive electrode) is properly placed on the patient prior to the start of surgery. Plug the patient ground pad into the machine (most newer machines will not allow the machine to activate in monopolar mode unless the grounding pad is plugged in).
- Fire safety precautions must be followed. These include:
  - Allow all prep solutions to dry completely before using the ESU.
  - Use a special endotracheal tube if electrosurgery will be performed near the airway.
  - Use flame-retardant drapes.
  - When not using the handpiece, place it back in the holder; DO NOT place it on dry drapes or towels.
  - Oxygen should be delivered at the lowest possible concentration.

- Water or saline must be available on the surgical field (usually on the back table).
- Portable fire extinguishers must be readily available (halon extinguishers are recommended).
- Nonflammable anesthetics must be used.
- During anorectal procedures, the rectum must be packed with a sterile water-soaked sponge to prevent a methane gas fire.
- NEVER turn off or disable alarms. Do not turn the volume too low; personnel should be able to hear the "beeping sound" when the electrode is activated. This sounds alerts all personnel that the tip is activated (hot).
- Use an instrument (not your hands!) to change the electrode tip.
- Do not loop the cords around metal devices or instruments.
- Make sure all jewelry is removed from the patient prior to surgery. Metal jewelry can act as a conductor and cause alternate-site burns.
- If the patient has a pacemaker or an implanted defibrillator, consult the cardiologist before surgery to find out whether or not the device needs to be shut off.
- DO NOT allow patient to come in contact with metal surfaces on the OR bed.
- Suction smoke and plume during electrosurgery use (a smoke evacuation system is recommended rather than just regular suctioning).

What to Do If the Patient Sustains a Burn

If a patient is burned and the electrosurgical device might have been the cause (e.g., you remove the grounding pad and the patient's skin underneath the pad is burned), this falls under federal mandatory reporting laws. What does staff need to do?

- Notify the surgeon immediately that a burn has occurred and have him or her look at the area. The surgeon will need to talk to the patient about what happened and may need to order treatment (e.g., ointments or dressings) for the burn.
- Document the facts of how the skin looks in the patient's perioperative record. Document that the surgeon was notified and what was done to treat the burn area.
- Save ALL disposable parts of the electrosurgical unit used on that patient, including the grounding pad, electrosurgical pencil and tips. Put these supplies in a bag and send them with the machine to biomedical engineering to be checked.
- The electrosurgical machine should NOT be used on any other patient until it has been checked and cleared by biomedical engineering.
- Notify your supervisor (who in turn needs to notify risk management). Fill out your institution's quality assurance paperwork (usually known as an *incidence* or *variance report*).

Troubleshooting Tips

As with any device, troubleshooting starts with the seemingly obvious and simple:

- Make sure the machine is plugged in.
- Make sure the machine is turned on.
- Check to see that the machine is in "ready" mode, not "standby."

After checking that the three troubleshooting tasks are done, start to look for the problem.

PROBLEM	WHAT TO LOOK AT
When the surgeon presses the button, the handpiece doesn't work.	■ Is the handpiece plugged into the proper place? ■ Is the handpiece plugged in all the way (snuggly)? ■ Is the grounding pad plugged into the machine? ■ Is there a problem with the grounding pad (has it lifted off the skin, folded on itself or torn)?
The grounding pad light is lit up.	■ Is the grounding pad plugged into the machine? ■ Has the grounding pad begun to lift off the patient's skin? ■ Is there a kink or tear in the grounding pad cord? ■ Has the grounding pad torn or folded (especially if the grounding pad was applied prior to positioning)?
I turn the machine "on" but the power doesn't come on.	■ Is the machine plugged in? ■ Is the cord kinked or frayed? If the cord is frayed or split, do not use this machine — get another one. ■ Try another electrical outlet (sometimes there is a problem with power to one outlet). ■ If the machine is plugged in and you've tried other outlets without any luck, get another machine and have biomedical engineering check out the problem machine.

■ The supervisor and/or risk management department will report the incident to the proper federal reporting agency following your institution's policy.

MEDICAL GASES

There are six common medical gases used in the OR: oxygen, nitrogen, nitrous oxide, carbon dioxide, helium and argon. Each gas has a specific purpose and a mix-up could be *disastrous*.

The Food and Drug Administration (FDA) recommends that each medical gas be stored in a cylinder of a specific color to make identification easier and a mix-up less likely. DO NOT rely solely on the cylinder color; *read the label on the cylinder carefully!* The regulator for the cylinder is another safety feature. Regulators are gas-specific and are not interchangeable; never modify a gas regulator from one type of gas to try to make it fit another.

These pages contain pictures and descriptions of each gas as well as specific safety tips. At the end of this section, general safety tips for handling medical gases are presented.

General Medical Gas Cylinder Safety

Medical gases are the only ones that have a regulated color system for the cylinders. Although it is *never* recommended that you rely on cylinder color alone *(read the label!)*, here are the FDA cylinder color recommendations to help with identification:

- **Air:** yellow
- **Carbon dioxide:** gray
- **Cyclopropane:** orange
- **Helium:** brown
- **Nitrogen:** black
- **Nitrous oxide:** blue
- **Oxygen:** green

General Guidelines for the Safe Handling of Medical Gas Cylinders

1. Read the label! Know what you are using before you use it. Never use an unmarked cylinder or one bearing a label that is unreadable.

2. Store cylinders away from flammable material. Do not use oily or greasy substances to clean the cylinders.

3. Store cylinders in an upright position and make sure that they are secured at all times. Use handcarts to transport cylinders. Do not allow cylinders to hit against one another.

4. Store cylinders away from sources of heat or electricity.

5. Do not try to modify regulators from one type of gas to fit another type of gas cylinder. *Remember:* Regulators are gas-specific and NOT interchangeable!

6. Store all cylinders in a well-ventilated area.

7. Let the experts do any repairs that are necessary. Do not try to repair damaged cylinders, regulators or gauges.

8. Never use a cylinder that is damaged or has a damaged pressure gauge or regulator.

Name: oxygen

Alias: O_2

Medication Class: essential gas

Use: provides supplemental oxygen to organs and tissue

Features: can be given via cannula, mask or Ambu bag; a flow rate for cannula should be 1 to 3 L; a flow rate of 8 to 10 L is best for mask; a flow rate of 10 to 15 L is needed for an Ambu bag

Additional Information: liter flow dependant on which vehicle the oxygen is being delivered by (cannula, mask, Ambu bag, and so on)

- **Cylinder Color:** green
- **Safety Tips:** flammable: caution must be taken when using the ESU or laser in areas where oxygen concentration may be high (e.g., the face or neck or under drapes)

Nitrous oxide

Name: nitrous oxide

Alias: none

Medication Class: inhalation anesthetic

Use: used in conjunction with other agents to provide balanced anesthesia; can be used in specific circumstances to create a pneumoperitoneum

Features: has little effect on heart rate or blood pressure; not potent enough to be used alone for general anesthesia

Additional Information: gas diffuses into closed spaces thus making it contraindicated for some surgeries (e.g., tympanoplasty)

- **Cylinder Color:** blue
- **Safety Tips:** nonflammable but does support combustion; use ESU or laser with caution in areas where high concentrations are likely (e.g., face or neck)

Name: nitrogen

Alias: none

Use: provides pneumatic power to equipment such as saws, drills, bone cement mixers and irrigators

Features: nonflammable

Additional Information:

- **Cylinder Color:** black
- **Safety Tips:** make sure all connections to equipment are secure

Name: carbon dioxide

Alias: CO_2

Use: insufflates the abdomen during laparoscopic surgery; used in cryosurgery

Features: odorless; does not support combustion; readily absorbed by the body

Additional Information: has the potential to cause hypercarbia leading to metabolic acidosis

- **Cylinder Color:** gray
- **Safety Tips:** monitor patient for signs of respiratory or cardiac problems (signs of acidosis due to break down of carbon dioxide into carbolic acid)

Name: Argon

Alias: none

Use: argon beam coagulation

Features: colorless; odorless; nonflammable; when ionized by electricity the argon provides an efficient pathway for the current to travel on

Additional Information:

- **Cylinder Color:** teal
- **Safety Tips:** a grounding pad must be placed on the patient before using argon beam coagulation (electrical current is passing through the patient)

Name: helium

Alias: none

Use: anesthesia; used with at least 21% oxygen to assist with flow of oxygen into the alveoli and prevent atelectasis (used in patients with severe respiratory obstruction as an oxygen carrier)

Features: colorless, odorless, nonflammable

Additional Information:

- **Cylinder Color:** brown
- **Safety Tips:** asphyxia can result if given with less than 21% oxygen; can diffuse through tubing if rubber tubing is used

PNEUMATIC TOURNIQUET

The pneumatic tourniquet is used to create a bloodless surgical area by limiting circulation to a patient's operative limb. Sometimes, it can be used in the administration of regional anesthesia. This device is used for procedures involving the knee, lower leg, ankle, foot, distal humerus, elbow, forearm, wrist and hand.

The tourniquet cuff is an air bladder surrounded by a nylon cover (see Fig. 1-82A), similar to a blood pressure cuff. It is placed proximal to the surgical site. Cuffs are available in sizes ranging from 8 to 42 inches.

Before applying the tourniquet cuff, check the skin for breaks or lesions and then pad the area circumferentially with Webril and stockinette. The padding helps to prevent undo pinching or damage to the skin. Once the padding is applied and smoothed (it should not have wrinkles that could dig into the skin when the tourniquet is inflated), the tourniquet cuff is applied around the entire circumference of the limb and fastened snuggly in place (see Fig. 1-83). It is hooked to the inflation machine tubing. The limb is then exsanguinated using an Esmarch bandage (see Fig. 1-82B). Once the limb has been exsanguinated, the cuff can be inflated. The surgeon is the one who decides at what point the cuff should be inflated and de-

FIGURE 1-83 Padded tourniquet applied to leg.

flated. The circulating nurse must note the time of inflation and deflation in his or her documentation.

The tourniquet is inflated using a machine that pumps compressed gas into the cuff. Generally, the surgeon will tell the circulator at what inflation pressure he or she wants the tourniquet set, based on patient systolic blood pressure, but there are some general safety guidelines for inflation pressures.

There are several pneumatic tourniquets available, each having a slightly different control panel. Although they may look different, each machine's control panel (see Fig. 1-84) has similar functions. Most machines can have two separate cuffs connected to them simultaneously, allowing for placement of the cuffs on two extremities (e.g., bilateral knee replacements) at the beginning of the procedure rather than trying to remove the cuff from one extremity and apply it to another in the middle of a procedure. Each cuff is attached to a separate set of tubing and controlled by a separate set of controls. Only one cuff is inflated at a time. The timer is reset when the first cuff is deflated and the second one inflated.

The control panel includes these buttons: power on/off switch, inflate and deflate buttons for each cuff and buttons to increase and decrease cuff pressure. Located on the front of the machine is a display of inflation time and cuff inflation pressure.

FIGURE 1-82 A) Tourniquet cuff. B) Esmarch bandage.

WATCH OUT!	Guidelines for Inflation Pressures

- Pressures for lower extremities should not exceed
- *Adult patient:* 100–150 mm Hg above the systolic blood pressure
- *Pediatric patient:* 100 mm Hg above the systolic blood pressure
- Pressure for upper extremities should not exceed 30–75 mm Hg above the patient's systolic blood pressure.

Inflation pressure recommendations may vary by device manufacturer. Make sure you know the manufacturer's recommendations for the device used in your institution.

FIGURE 1-84 A) Tourniquet machine. B) Control panel.

Tourniquet Safety

- Only personnel who are familiar with the use of the device should be using it. If you are unsure of how to use the device, read the manufacturer's instructions and seek help from someone who knows how to use the device.
- All staff who will be using the device need to demonstrate ongoing competency in its use.
- Policies and procedures must be in place regarding device use.
- Tourniquets should be applied only by *licensed* personnel (registered nurse, surgeon, physician assistant)
- The limb where the tourniquet cuff will be placed must be assessed by the circulator before cuff application and after cuff removal at the end of the procedure. Both of these assessments must be documented in the patient record.

- Document the time from inflation of the cuff to deflation of the cuff (known as "tourniquet time") in the patient record
- If the procedure requires that the tourniquet remain inflated longer than the recommended times, deflate the tourniquet for 10 minutes then re-inflate. This allows circulation to be restored to the area and decreases the risk of damage.
- Make efforts to ensure prep solutions do not seep underneath the tourniquet or into the padding. Fluid pooling under the tourniquet could cause tissue damage such as burns.
- If the tourniquet appears to be malfunctioning, use another one and have biomedical engineering check the one that is malfunctioning. Repairs should be done by qualified personnel only.
- As with any electrical device, check all cords for fraying, cracks or exposed wire prior to use. If any of these things are found, DO NOT use the device.
- Check tubing that connects the cuff to the machine prior to use for cracks or holes. Check connections to make sure there are not any leaks.
- Most cuffs are designed for single patient use and are discarded after the procedure. Machines and tubing need to be decontaminated according to manufacturer's instructions and institutional policy.
- Do not disable or make inaudible the time or pressure alarms. They are there for patient safety and need to remain audible to personnel.

WATCH OUT! | **Tourniquet Time Guidelines**

- *Upper extremity:* the tourniquet may remain inflated up to 60 minutes
- *Lower extremity:* the tourniquet may remain inflated 60–120 minutes

Tourniquet times exceeding these limits increase the chance of nerve damage, tissue necrosis and damage to blood vessels. Check your institution's policies regarding maximum tourniquet time allowed.

AUTOTRANSFUSION

Autotransfusion is the reinfusion of the patient's own blood or blood products. Thse products may be donated prior to surgery, or blood may be collected intraoperatively or postoperatively and then reinfused. It is the intraoperative and postoperative blood collection and reinfusion devices that are covered in this section.

Why Reinfuse?

Autotransfusion is sometimes preferable to a donor transfusion because it eliminates the danger of blood incompatibility and possible disease transmission. In some cases, patients who refuse a blood transfusion from an outside source may be willing to accept an autotransfusion.

There are times when you should not collect the patient's blood and reinfuse it:

- If the patient has a known infection (localized or systemic)
- If the blood has been exposed to antibiotics (including antibiotic irrigating solutions) or collagen hemostatic agents; this can cause blood to coagulate in the machine
- If the blood has mixed with amniotic fluid or gastric or bowel contents

Several types of devices can be used to collect blood, process it and ready it for reinfusion back into the patient. The following sections describe the most common types of machines and their uses.

Cell Saver or Cell Salvager

The cell saver or cell salvager allows the blood to be suctioned directly from the surgical field into the machine (see Fig. 1-85). It can also suction bloody saline from a basin in which bloody sponges were immersed in saline. The machine filters and anti-coagulates the blood and fluid, readying it for IV reinfusion back to the patient. This process causes little or no harm to the red blood cells.

The cell saver is capable of processing large quantities of blood and irrigation fluid and is used when a large blood loss is possible, such as a ruptured spleen or large blood vessel, major spinal surgery, major orthopedic procedures or multiple trauma with suspected major bleeding.

One major disadvantage to the cell saver device is that it may require a dedicated operator to run it. Check your institution's policy regarding who can operate a cell saver.

OrthoPat Blood Salvaging Device

This blood salvaging device is designed for use during orthopedic procedures in which blood loss may be sufficient to require transfusion (e.g., total hip replacement). The blood is suctioned

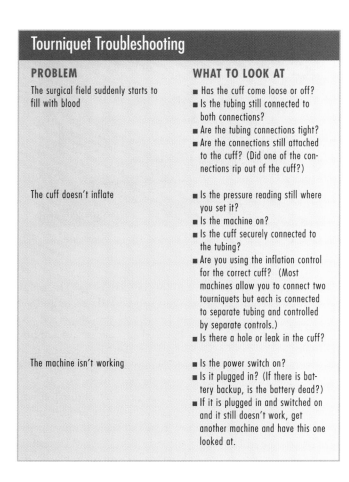

Tourniquet Troubleshooting

PROBLEM	WHAT TO LOOK AT
The surgical field suddenly starts to fill with blood	■ Has the cuff come loose or off? ■ Is the tubing still connected to both connections? ■ Are the tubing connections tight? ■ Are the connections still attached to the cuff? (Did one of the connections rip out of the cuff?)
The cuff doesn't inflate	■ Is the pressure reading still where you set it? ■ Is the machine on? ■ Is the cuff securely connected to the tubing? ■ Are you using the inflation control for the correct cuff? (Most machines allow you to connect two tourniquets but each is connected to separate tubing and controlled by separate controls.) ■ Is there a hole or leak in the cuff?
The machine isn't working	■ Is the power switch on? ■ Is it plugged in? (If there is battery backup, is the battery dead?) ■ If it is plugged in and switched on and it still doesn't work, get another machine and have this one looked at.

FIGURE 1-85 Cell saver machine.

from the surgical field into the machine where it is cleansed, anticoagulated and collected in a bag for IV reinfusion.

The OrthoPat (see Fig. 1-86) can be used postoperatively to collect and prepare blood for reinfusion. Instead of suctioning blood from the surgical field, the OrthoPat device is attached to the drain. The blood is drained from the surgical wound into the machine and cleansed and prepared for reinfusion.

This device is capable of processing smaller amounts of blood and fluid than a cell saver and is designed for use in orthopedic procedures where blood loss is intermittent. It is *not* designed to be used for major blood loss such as with a ruptured spleen or bleeding aorta. One major advantage is that the machine is fully automated and can be monitored by the circulating personnel. It does not require a dedicated operator.

Autotransfusion Drains

The simplest of autotransfusion devices are the postoperative collection drains (see Fig. 1-87). These devices are closed collection systems that use a three-spring evacuator (similar to a Hemovac drain) or controlled wall suction to suction blood from the surgical wound postoperatively and collect it for possible reinfusion. These devices contain filters within the collection chamber to filter out clots and debris. They have access ports to allow for the addition of anticoagulant medication.

The advantages to these drains are that they are easy to set up and use, they are closed systems, thus decreasing the chance of staff exposure to blood, and they are relatively inexpensive

FIGURE 1-87 A) and B) Postoperative autotransfusion drains.

FIGURE 1-86 OrthoPat machine.

when compared with other reinfusion technology. The transfer of the fluid into the reinfusion bag is easily accomplished (usually the push of a button or lever), and you only need one device per patient (they can be used to collect and reinfuse multiple times). The disadvantages are that they can be used postoperatively only (not intraoperatively), and they have a smaller collection capacity than some other devices.

As with any medical device, no matter which autotransfusion technology is being used you must make sure you are familiar with the device and how to use it *prior* to using it on your patient. If you are unfamiliar with the device, check your institution's procedure for its use and the manufacturer's instructions.

PATIENT POSITIONING EQUIPMENT

Name: gel pad
Alias: none
Use: intraoperatively pads pressure points (e.g., heels, ankles, knees, elbows, hands)
Features: contain a gel substance that supports the area without placing pressure on it
Additional Information: available in many sizes and firmnesses

Name: chest rolls
Alias: none
Use: lift the chest off the stretcher during prone positioning to allow for chest expansion during respiration
Features: padded; contains a gel substance for softness
Additional Information: available in many sizes and firmnesses; should be placed so that it extends from the top of the chest to the waist

Name: bean bag positioner
Alias: none
Use: stabilizes the torso in lateral positioning
Features: air is taken out of the bean bag using suction to firm the bag and hold the patient in place
Additional Information: air is suctioned out after the patient is positioned

Name: Shea headrest
Alias: none
Use: positions the head during supine or lateral positioning
Features: made of foam to cushion head
Additional Information: available in adult and pediatric sizes

Name: elbow gel pad
Alias: none
Use: intraoperatively pads elbows
Features: has gel inside for padding; Velcro strap allows for secure fastening around the arm
Additional Information: available in several styles and sizes; can be strapped around the elbow or laid out straight with the elbow resting on the widest area

Name: stirrup holders

Alias: none

Use: attach stirrups or other positioning devices to the surgical bed

Features: attach onto OR table rails

Additional Information: come in many sizes and styles

Name: lateral hip post

Alias: none

Use: supports the lateral aspect of the thigh during orthopedic surgery

Features: padded support area, post is solid; to adjust height, slide up or down in the stirrup holder

Additional Information: positioned using stirrup holder attached to the OR bed rail

Name: gentle touch headrest

Alias: none

Use: supports the head and airway while the patient is in the prone position

Features: soft padding for face (white side is placed toward patient face); cut out area for positioning of the endotracheal tube

Additional Information: comes vacuum sealed; needs to be taken out of the package and allowed to "puff up" prior to use

Name: prone view positioner

Alias: none

Use: supports head and airway while the patient is in the prone position

Features: mirrored bottom allows for viewing of patient airway; foam padding is placed inside the rigid support

Additional Information: use only the prone view padding with the prone view positioner; padding is single patient use, rigid support is disinfected between patients

Name: Opti-Gard eye protector

Alias: none

Use: protects patient's eyes while patient is in the prone position

Features: padding on the borders of the glasses with rigid plastic eye shields keeps the eyes from being compressed while the patient is prone

Additional Information: none

Name: wrist support

Alias: arm strap

Use: supports the arm to help prevent it from falling off the arm board intraoperatively

Features: can be made of various material; Velcro is easy to put on and take off quickly

Additional Information: a towel, washcloth or other padding should be placed over the patient's wrist prior to applying the strap

Name: total knee stabilizer

Alias: none

Use: supports the foot while the leg is flexed (e.g., during total knee arthroplasty)

Features: padded to protect the sole of the foot

Additional Information: available in several styles; foot pad is replaceable

Name: axillary roll

Alias: none

Use: helps avoid pressure on the axillary nerves and blood vessels during lateral positioning

Features: can be made from several readily available items such as rolled towel or blanket

Additional Information: an inflated blood pressure cuff or full IV bag also may be used

Name: pelvic positioner

Alias: none

Use: supports and holds the pelvic area in place during lateral positioning (e.g., during hip surgery)

Features: padded; attached to the OR table using stirrup holders

Additional Information: available in several styles

Name: safety belt

Alias: safety strap; restraint strap

Use: helps to keep the patient's legs secured in place during surgery

Features: some have Velcro straps for fastening whereas others have buckles; available in various lengths

Additional Information: the belt should be placed approximately 2 inches above the patient's knees; the strap should be snug but not tight (you should be able to slip two fingers under the belt)

Name: hand positioner

Alias: none

Use: holds fingers spread for surgery on the palm

Features: can be adjusted to hold one or all fingers; padded with foam to cushion the hand

Additional Information: single patient use

MISCELLANEOUS EQUIPMENT

Name: sharps container

Alias: none

Use: safe disposal of all contaminated sharps (e.g., needles, blades, trocars)

Features: puncture proof; marked with biohazardous waste symbol

Additional Information: available in a variety of sizes

Name: ultrasonic cleaner

Alias: none

Use: cleans debris from delicate instruments (e.g., eye instruments); cleaning debris from hard to reach places on instruments (e.g., box locks, serrations)

Features: *cavitation* is used to remove the debris, in other words, high-frequency sound waves are converted to vibrations, which create bubbles and cause the bubbles to *implode* (collapse inward); the implosion of the bubbles creates a vacuum that pulls debris from the instruments

Additional Information: instruments made of dissimilar metals should not be placed in the ultrasonic cleaner together; gross debris must be removed from instruments before placing them in the ultrasonic cleaner; various models are available; models can contain one to three chambers

Name: sequential compression device

Alias: SCD

Use: helps to prevent venous stasis and decrease the chance of thrombus formation

Features: stockings massage the legs in an upward pattern to help prevent pooling of blood in the lower extremities

Additional Information: stockings are available in small, medium, large and extra large sizes

Name: head light

Alias: head lamp

Use: provides a concentrated area of light on the wound site for visualization by the surgeon during a procedure

Features: adjustable headpiece allows for snug fit to the surgeon's head; beam can be adjusted to the area the surgeon is viewing

Additional Information: available in many styles and sizes

Name: sponge collection bag

Alias: none

Use: separates used sponges for ease of count

Features: each holder has 10 individual compartments; see through front allows for ease of visualization of sponges

Additional Information: for ease and efficiency of counting, each type of sponge should be placed in a separate holder; do not "mix" different types (e.g., lap pads and RayTecs) in the same holder

Name: smoke evacuation system

Alias: none

Use: suctions and filters surgical plume

Features: system contains HEPA filters and absorbers to trap surgical plume

Additional Information: nozzle tip must be within 2 inches of the surgical site in order to be effective; filter and tubing must be changed between patients; filters are considered biohazardous waste

Name: C-arm

Alias: image intensifier

Use: intraoperative fluoroscopy

Features: image is immediately available to view; C-arm can be manipulated to give multiple views of the operative site

Additional Information: personnel need to wear lead aprons or stand behind a lead shield when C-arm is in use; C-arm is draped with a sterile C-arm drape

Name: mini C-arm

Alias: image intensifier

Use: intraoperative fluoroscopy; used primarily for imaging fingers, hands, wrists or knees

Features: smaller and more easily maneuvered than conventional C-arms; exposes patients and staff to less radiation

Additional Information: lead apron should be worn when operating the machine (special lighter mini C-arm lead is available in some institutions); C-arm is draped with sterile C-arm cover; machine can be operated by the surgeon using a foot pedal

Name: fire extinguisher

Alias: none

Use: extinguishes small fires

Features: pin must be pulled in order to operate extinguisher; there are several models available, each one specific to certain types of fire; make sure you use the correct extinguisher for the type of material that has ignited

Additional Information: most ORs are equipped with multi-purpose (ABC) extinguishers that can be used on most materials; only use the extinguisher if the fire is small and you have been properly trained in extinguisher use

Name: Doppler

Alias: none

Use: assesses blood flow through a blood vessel before, during and after surgery

Features: sterile probe should be available if intra-operative use is expected

Additional Information: available in many models and styles

Name: Mayfield instrument table

Alias: overhead table

Use: holds instruments and supplies during craniotomy or spine procedures

Features: provides a large work area for the scrub person (33.5- × 42-inch surface)

Additional Information: draped with an overhead table drape; can be draped continuously with the patient to produce a single large sterile field

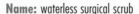

Name: surgical scrub brush

Alias: none

Use: performing the surgical scrub prior to entering the surgical suite

Features: soft foam side for performing skin scrub, bristle side for performing fingernail scrub

Additional Information: available with hexachlorophene or povidone-iodine (Betadine) soap impregnated in the brush

Name: waterless surgical scrub

Alias: several brand names: Avagard, Triseptin

Use: performing the surgical scrub prior to entering the surgical suite

Features: does not require the use of water; non-abrasive to the skin; has built-in emollient to control drying out of the skin

Additional Information: follow manufacturer's instructions for use; use only the amount the manufacturer recommends and the procedure they suggest; procedures vary for each type of scrub

Surgical Session Review

1) All of the following are true about masks *except:*
  a. they should be changed after each case
  b. they protect the wearer from spraying of blood/body fluids
  c. they have to be worn in unrestricted areas of the OR
  d. they must be worn so that they cover the mouth and the nose

2) Which of the following statements is *false* regarding OR attire:
  a. caps or hats must cover all hair (including facial hair)
  b. cloth caps or hats can be worn for 3 consecutive days without laundering
  c. tunic style scrub tops should be tucked into your scrub pants
  d. Regular eyeglasses alone do not meet the standards for protective eyewear

3) Unsterile personnel should stand a *minimum* of _____ inches from the sterile field.
  a. 6-8
  b. 12-18
  c. 20-24
  d. 24-28

4) Principles of aseptic technique include:
  a. keep talking at the field to a minimum
  b. only sterile (scrubbed) personnel handle sterile items
  c. create the sterile field as close to the time of surgery as possible
  d. all of the above

5) All of the following are true about sterile drapes *except:*
  a. they should be made of a low-linting material
  b. once in place, they should not be moved
  c. handling should be kept to a minimum
  d. the part of the drape that falls below the level of the table top is sterile

6) The maximum continuous time that a tourniquet should be left inflated on a leg is _____ minutes.
  a. 30
  b. 60
  c. 90
  d. 120

7) Which of the following might be used to position a patient who is undergoing surgery on the lower back?
  a. Jackson table
  b. Wilson frame
  c. Andrews frame
  d. all of the above

8) A horseshoe, Mayfield or Shea may be used to position the patient's _____.
  a. head
  b. arm
  c. foot
  d. shoulders

9) Arms should NEVER be extended more than _____ degrees on an arm board.
  a. 45
  b. 65
  c. 90
  d. 120

10) Hyperextension of the arm can cause damage to the:
  a. peroneal nerve
  b. popliteal nerve
  c. brachial plexus
  d. chordae tendineae

11) All of the following are types of stirrups *except:*
  a. candy cane
  b. boot
  c. knee release
  d. knee crutch

12) A _____ is one of the most common types of suction tip used to clear the airway.
  a. Yankauer
  b. Neuro
  c. Frasier
  d. Poole

13) Which of the following types of electrosurgery unit *does not* require the use of a grounding pad?
  a. monopolar
  b. argon beam
  c. bipolar
  d. all of the above require a grounding pad

14) Fire safety rules during the use of electrosurgery include:
  a. allow all prep solutions to dry completely
  b. water or saline must be available on the surgical field
  c. when not in use, the handpiece should be placed back in a holder
  d. all of the above

15) In reference to electrosurgery units, ABC stands for:
  a. aluminum beam coagulation
  b. argon beam coagulation
  c. argon beam cautery
  d. aluminum beam cautery

16) Which of the following staff members should *not* apply the pneumatic tourniquet?
a. surgeon
b. physician assistant
c. registered nurse
d. surgical technologist

17) Ultrasonic cleaners use _____ to remove debris from instruments.
a. cavitation
b. steam
c. ethylene oxide
d. Cidex

18) _____ is an anesthetic gas.
a. oxygen
b. nitrogen
c. nitrous oxide
d. argon

19) An Optigard protector is used when the patient is prone to protect his or her _____.
a. fingers
b. hands
c. toes
d. eyes

20) A Doppler is used to assess _____ flow.
a. urine
b. coronary artery
c. blood
d. brain wave

CHAPTER 2
General Surgical Supplies

SURGICAL SPONGES

Surgical sponges come in a variety of shapes and sizes, each with its own specific purpose. The most common uses for surgical sponges are to absorb blood and fluid. They also can be used as padding to protect tissue from retractor blades, to wipe debris from instruments or to perform blunt tissue dissection.

Sponges intended for use inside of the body cavity share several characteristics:

- Lint-free
- Soft, to avoid damaging tissue
- Radiopaque strip sewn into them (to make them visible on x-ray if left inside a wound)

Depending on your institution, various sponges are referred to by names other than what are listed in this section. I have chosen to go with the commonly accepted names for the various sponges.

General Sponge Handling Tips

- Sponges are contaminated with blood or body fluids. Use Standard Precautions.
- Gloves must be worn when handling sponges. Never use your bare hands.
- Sponges should be tossed off the field into a proper receptacle (e.g., kick bucket or basin), not onto the floor or into the trash.
- When setting up your table preoperatively, like sponges should be kept together and separate from other types (e.g., all laparotomy sponges in one area of the table, all RayTec sponges in another area) to avoid confusion and to make counting more efficient.
- Soiled sponges should be separated to keep all like sponges together. If using a clear sponge counting bag, do not mix different sponges in the same bag; use a separate sponge bag for each type of sponge.
- Keep small sponges, such as cherries or dissectors, attached to a clamp or in the holder. Do not leave them loose on your table or Mayo stand. These sponges are very small and could easily be lost (or fall inside the wound).
- To avoid damaging tissue, moisten sponges that are being used inside the chest, abdomen or pelvis with saline before use.
- Once the initial count has been done, never remove a sponge from the operating room (OR).
- When counting sponges, separate each sponge to avoid missing a sponge or miscounting. Each type of sponge should be counted separately.

RayTec

The RayTec sponge is a 4 × 4-inch sponge with a radiopaque strip sewn into it. It is made of loosely woven gauze, which gives it a rough surface (see Fig. 2-1). These sponges are used when the incision is small. Loose RayTecs are generally not allowed on the field during a laparotomy because they could easily be lost in the abdominopelvic cavity. Instead, the large laparotomy sponge is used.

Wrapped around the fingers, RayTecs can be used for blunt tissue dissection. They can be mounted on a sponge stick and used to absorb fluid or dissect tissue inside the abdominal cavity. Moistened with saline or sterile water, they are often used to keep surgical instruments free of debris.

Caution must be taken NOT to mix up RayTecs with 4 × 4-inch gauze dressing sponges because they look very similar. The important difference is that dressing sponges DO NOT have the radiopaque strip sewn into them and therefore could easily be lost in the wound. Depending on the institution, dressing sponges are either kept in an area separate from the Raytec sponges being used during the procedure or they are not introduced onto the sterile field until the wound is closed.

RayTec sponges come in a package of 10. RayTecs should be separated and counted individually (not in groups of 2 or 3) to ensure an accurate count.

FIGURE 2-1 RayTec sponge with radiopaque strip and plain dressing sponge.

Laparotomy Sponges

Laparotomy sponges, known as *laps,* are used when large incisions of the thoracic or abdominopelvic cavity are involved, during vascular surgery involving large blood vessels or during major orthopedic cases (see Fig. 2-2). These sponges are most commonly used for the absorption of large amounts of blood or body fluid. Moistened with saline, they can be used as padding between body tissue and retractors to decrease the chance of tissue injury. Laparotomy pads also may be used to wipe debris from instruments.

Laparotomy sponges measure 12 × 12 inches or 18 × 18 inches. They are made of surgical cotton and have a radiopaque strip sewed onto them. They come in packages of five. When counting laparotomy sponges, separate and count each one individually.

Laparotomy Tape

Laparotomy tape is a long, thin laparotomy sponge. Made of surgical cotton, it measures 4 × 18 inches and has a radiopaque strip sewn onto it (see Fig. 2-3). These sponges are used to absorb blood or body fluid from a narrow, deep incision (e.g., lumbar spinal surgery). Laparotomy tapes come in packages of five.

Tonsil (Round) Sponges

Tonsil sponges are round pieces of cotton covered with gauze that have a string attached for easy retrieval from the throat. They have a radiopaque strip sewn into them (see Fig. 2-4). Typically these sponges are mounted on a clamp (e.g., Pean) and placed in the throat to control bleeding in the tonsil bed. They can be used plain, or they can have a hemostatic agent applied to them. When you remove the sponges from the throat, it is important to make sure that you have *both* the sponge and the string because a string could get cut during the procedure. Tonsil sponges come in packages of five.

Peanuts

Peanuts, also known as *dissectors, pushers* and *Kitners,* are small oval pieces of cotton wrapped in gauze. A radiopaque strip is sewn in (see Fig. 2-5). These sponges can be used to absorb small amounts of blood or fluid but are used more commonly for blunt tissue dissection. Peanuts are always mounted on a

FIGURE 2-3 Laparotomy tape. Notice placement of the blue radiopaque strip.

FIGURE 2-4 Tonsil sponges.

FIGURE 2-2 Laparotomy sponge. Notice placement of the blue radiopaque strip.

FIGURE 2-5 Peanuts sponges.

clamp (e.g., Pean) for use. They should never be allowed to be loose on the field, table or Mayo stand due to their small size; they easily could be lost into the wound. Peanuts come five to a package.

Cherries

Cherry sponges are small, round balls of tightly wrapped cotton tape with a radiopaque center. They may look similar to a peanut but are more tightly wrapped and stiffer (see Fig. 2-6). These sponges are used for blunt tissue dissection. Cherries are always mounted on a clamp (e.g., Pean) for use. They should never be allowed to be loose on the field, table or Mayo stand due to their small size; they easily could be lost into the wound. Cherries come five to a package.

Neurosurgical Sponges

A neurosurgical sponge, also known as a *patty* or *cottonoid,* is a flat, square or rectangular sponge made of cotton or synthetic material with a radiopaque strip down the center (see Fig. 2-7). The sponge has a string attached for easy retrieval. These sponges come in a variety of sizes, ranging from ⅛- to 1-inch wide and ⅛ to 6 inches long.

Neurosurgical sponges are used for hemostasis during neurosurgery, but they also can be used during vascular or ear/nose procedures. They are moistened with either saline or thrombin prior to being placed on the tissue. Larger rectangular sponges can be moistened with a topical anesthetic (e.g., liquid cocaine) and inserted into the nose prior to nasal procedures. These sponges can be placed over an area to be suctioned and a small suction placed on top of them instead of directly on the tissue, thus protecting the tissue from damage.

To keep the sponges sorted and easily accessible, they are moistened with saline and mounted on a flat, metal or plastic tray called a *patty tray.* The sponges are passed to the surgeon mounted on a pair of smooth jawed forceps (e.g., bayonet forceps). When receiving the sponge back from the surgeon, make sure you have *both* the sponge and the string; a string could get cut during the procedure. Neurosurgical sponges come in packages of 10.

Eye Sponges

Eye sponges, also known as *spears,* are small, flat triangular pieces of cellulose each mounted on a small, thin piece of plastic (see Fig. 2-8). These sponges are used to absorb small amounts of blood and fluid during eye procedures or some microsurgeries. They do not have a radiopaque strip because they are not used inside a body cavity. Eye sponges come in packages of 10.

FIGURE 2-7 Neurosurgical sponges.

FIGURE 2-6 Cherries sponges.

FIGURE 2-8 Eye sponge.

HEMOSTATISTICS

Name: hemoclips

Alias: clips

Use: clip vessels or ducts

Features: available in sizes small (red cartridge), medium (blue cartridge) or large (orange cartridge)

Additional Information: clips may be metal or plastic; color of cartridge corresponds to the handle color of the applier; cartridges may be included as part of the count (not the individual clips)

Name: Gelfoam

Alias: absorbable gelatin sponge; Surgifoam

Use: hemostatic

Features: dry; applied topically; absorbable

Additional Information: available in a variety of sizes; can be cut up for use in small areas

Name: oxidized cellulose

Alias: Surgicel; Oxycel

Use: hemostatic

Features: absorbable; sheet can be cut to size needed; flexible

Additional Information: handle with dry forceps; comes in a variety of sheet sizes

Name: bone wax

Alias: none

Use: stopping bleeding on the bone surface

Features: pliable; can be molded to size and shape needed

Additional Information: can be applied by hand or with an instrument; store away from heat

Name: Avitene

Alias: microfibrillar collagen

Use: hemostatic

Features: absorbable; can be broken up into small pieces if necessary

Additional Information: should be handled with dry forceps; available in several sizes

Name: Collastat

Alias: collagen sponge

Use: hemostatic

Features: absorbable; comes as a sheet; sponge can be cut to desired size

Additional Information: handle with dry forceps; available in several sizes

Name: Gelfoam sterile powder

Alias: none

Use: hemostatic

Features: mixed with sterile saline and then applied

Additional Information: after mixing with sterile saline it can be shaped and applied to the desired surface

Name: silver nitrate sticks

Alias: none

Use: hemostatic

Features: when moistened (e.g., by blood from a bleeding vessel), the silver nitrate is activated and cauterizes the area

Additional Information: come in a canister to protect them from moisture; for use on small areas

Name: Surgicel fibrillar

Alias: oxidized cellulose (fiber)

Use: hemostatic

Features: can be torn or cut into desired size; fiber construction

Additional Information: comes in several sizes

Name: Thrombin, topical

Alias: none

Use: topical hemostasis; apply only to the surface of bleeding area; often Gelfoam (Surgifoam) is soaked in it and applied to bleeding

Features: comes as a powder; must be mixed with enclosed container of normal saline

Additional Information: available in 5000 U or 20,000 U vials or 20,000 U spray kit; must ONLY be used topically; CANNOT be injected

SYRINGES

Syringes are commonly used in the OR. Anesthesia care providers use them to measure and administer medication. Scrubbed personnel use syringes to measure and administer medications, measure and dispense irrigating solutions, withdraw fluid from body cavities and obtain liquid specimens to send for diagnosis. Circulators use syringes to measure and dispense medication to the field or administer medication to the patient. In these pages, the two major categories of syringes—those that you can place a needle onto and those that are used for irrigation—are be covered.

Syringes that have a tip where a needle can be placed come in many sizes and styles. Syringes are marked in milliliters (mL) or cubic centimeters (cc) for easy measurement. Milliliters and cubic centimeters are equivalent (1 mL = 1 cc). The most commonly used sizes are 1 mL, 3 mL, 5 mL, 10 mL, 12 mL, 20 mL and 60 mL. Which size you use depends on what you are using it for; a 1-mL syringe would be used to measure out small amounts of medication (e.g., pediatric dosages) whereas a 60-mL syringe might be used to withdraw large amounts of fluid from a patient's joint.

Despite the size differences among syringes, they all have the same basic components (see Fig. 2-9):

- Barrel
- Plunger
- Tip
- Measurement markings

Medication, solutions and fluids are drawn up into the syringe by holding the barrel and pulling back on the plunger until you have the desired amount in the barrel of the syringe.

To inject medication or solution, you hold the top of the barrel in your fingers and push down on the top of the plunger slowly and steadily until you have injected the desired amount.

Syringe Tips

There are two different types of syringe tips: Luer-Lok and plain (catheter tip; Luer-slip).

Luer-Lok Tip

As the name implies, the Luer-Lok tip (see Fig. 2-10) has threads; in order to place a needle on a Luer-Lok tip, you place the hub of the needle onto the tip and, with a twisting motion, lock it in place. You must twist the needle onto the tip in order to secure it. This is the most commonly used type of syringe.

Plain (Catheter Tip; Luer-slip) Tip

The plain tip syringe (see Fig. 2-11) does not have threads to lock the needle in place. The hub of the needle or end of a catheter is pushed onto the end of the tip.

Commonly used syringes are made of either plastic or glass. Plastic is by far the most common material used, but glass syringes are still available to be used for certain tasks (e.g., some anesthesia providers prefer glass syringes when inserting an epidural; some medication strengths could be affected by plastic) (see Fig. 2-12).

There are syringes available that have finger rings on the top of the barrel and plunger. These rings allow the user to insert fingers for better control of the rate of medication administration or force of irrigation. These are known as *three-ring, high-pressure* or *control syringes* (see Fig. 2-13).

FIGURE 2-10 Luer-Lok tip.

FIGURE 2-9 Parts of a syringe.

FIGURE 2-11 Plain catheter tip.

Tuberculin syringes and insulin syringes are both small syringes, but that is where the similarity ends. An insulin syringe should NEVER BE USED FOR ANYTHING OTHER THAN MEASURING AND ADMINISTERING INSULIN! The insulin syringe (see Fig. 2-14) is marked in *units of insulin* not milliliters (cubic centimeters) of volume. If you were to measure fluid or medication (other than insulin) in an insulin syringe, the measurement would be inaccurate and thus potentially dangerous. Only small dosages of medication should be drawn up using the tuberculin syringe (see Fig. 2-14).

Irrigating Syringes

In the OR, there are three common types of irrigating syringes: the Asepto, the bulb and the Toomey. These syringes are used to draw up and dispense irrigating solutions and do not have a needle placed on them.

Asepto Syringe

The Asepto syringe is the most common irrigating syringe found on the surgical field. It has a capacity of 120 mL. It has a bulb and barrel construction (see Fig. 2-15).

Bulb Syringe (Ear Syringe)

Most commonly thought of as a mechanism to remove fluid or mucus from an infant's nose or mouth, the bulb syringe can also be used for irrigation. In contrast to the Asepto, its construction is a bulb only (no barrel) (see Fig. 2-16). The bulb syringe is used to irrigate small incisions or delicate structures such as the brain or ears.

FIGURE 2–12 Glass syringe.

FIGURE 2–13 Three-ring, high-pressure or control syringe.

FIGURE 2–14 Tuberculin syringe: 1-mL capacity; marked in 0.1-mL increments (larger lines). Insulin syringe: marked in units of insulin (not mL).

FIGURE 2–15 Asepto syringe.

FIGURE 2–16 Bulb syringe.

Toomey Syringe

The Toomey syringe is used to irrigate or instill fluids into tubes or catheters. The plain style tip is long and tapered to fit inside the lumen of a catheter or tube. The Toomey has a capacity of 60 mL. The construction is the same as a regular syringe with a barrel and plunger but, unlike a regular syringe, the tip is designed to irrigate or instill fluids only; a needle cannot be placed on it (see Fig. 2-17).

Hypodermic Needles

Hypodermic needles are placed on the end of a syringe to allow medication to be drawn up into the syringe, to allow injection of fluid or medication into body tissue or to withdraw body fluid from tissues or joints. Small (fine) hypodermic needles may be used to remove small bits of tissue from biopsy needles.

Hypodermic needles are sized according to a numbering system. The important thing to remember is *the larger the number, the smaller the diameter of the needle.* The sizes of hypodermic needles range from 12 to 30 with a #12 having the largest diameter and a #30 having the smallest (see Fig. 2-18). Hypodermic needles range in length from ⅜ to 4 inches.

Regardless of the size or length of the hypodermic needle, they all have the same basic components (see Fig. 2-19):

- Hub
- Bevel
- Shaft

FIGURE 2–17 Toomey syringe.

FIGURE 2–18 Tip of 16-gauge needle and tip of a 27-gauge needle.

FIGURE 2–19 Parts of hypodermic needle.

Needle Safety

As with any sharp, hypodermic needles must be handled and disposed of with caution to avoid an inadvertent needlestick to yourself or other team member. Here are a few rules to follow to help promote safety when using needles:

- Know the location of your needles on the surgical field at all times.
- Attach or remove the needle from a syringe using a clamp or other instrument, NOT your hands.
- Never recap a needle using your hands; use the "scoop method" or a recapping device.
- Pass the syringe and needle using a "neutral zone"; avoid hand-to-hand passing when at all possible.
- Discard dirty needles by placing needle side down into a sharps holder (AccuCount or similar box). At the end of the case, discard the sharps holder into a puncture-proof sharps disposal bucket.
- If the needle is equipped with a safety shield, trigger the safety shield over the needle at the end of the case before disposing of it. *Remember:* On some needles, if you trigger the safety shield it cannot be retracted; therefore, the needle cannot be used again. That is why I recommend waiting until the end of the case to trigger the device.

SURGICAL WOUND DRESSINGS

A surgical dressing is placed over the surgical wound site immediately after the incision is closed. The main purpose of the dressing is to protect the surgical incision from contaminants in the environment, but dressings also can give the wound extra support, protect it from trauma, provide skin closure, apply pressure, débride it or absorb drainage.

Surgical dressings are placed over a fresh incision; therefore, they must be sterile to protect the wound from microbial contamination. When applying the dressing, it should be handled by the edges to avoid contaminating the part being placed over the wound. If the person applying the dressing has been wearing two pairs of sterile gloves during the procedure, the

Dressing materials do NOT have a radiopaque strip because they are not intended for use inside the body (see Fig. 2-20). Many dressing materials look similar to RayTec sponges and they easily could be confused. Dressing material should be kept in a separate area on the back table or not opened until the final surgical sponge count has been completed. Institution policy varies; check your institution's policies and procedures.

RayTec sponges should not be used as dressings. On a postoperative x-ray, the radiopaque strip would show up and could look like a RayTec sponge was left inside the patient.

FIGURE 2–21 2 × 2, 4 × 4 and drain sponges.

FIGURE 2–20 RayTec and 4 × 4 dressing sponge.

FIGURE 2–22 Abdominal dressing.

outer gloves should be removed before applying the dressing the dressing applied with the clean inner gloves.

Gauze Sponges

As the name implies, gauze sponges are squares of sterile gauze. They are the most common dressing used postoperatively. Gauze sponges are used mainly for protection of the wound and absorption of body fluids. These dressing are made to be low lint (to prevent lint from contaminating the wound) and absorbent and to wick blood and fluids into their layers to keep the wound dry. Gauze sponges come in a variety of sizes. The most common sizes are 4 × 4 inches and 2 × 2 inches (see Fig. 2-21). These sponges also may be referred to as *Toppers* or *Excilon sponges.*

Another type of gauze sponge is referred to as a *drain sponge*. A drain sponge is a 4 × 4-inch gauze sponge with a cross shape cut into it. The cross-shaped cutout is placed around the drain, allowing the dressing to fit snuggly and the drain to protrude.

Abdominal Dressing

The abdominal dressing (also known as the *ABD pad*) is a thick absorbent gauze dressing used to cover large wounds (see Fig. 2-22). The ABD pad can be used as a stand alone dressing or as an outer dressing when large amounts of

drainage are expected. These dressing are available in 5 × 9-inch and 8 × 10-inch sizes.

Eye Pad and Eye Shield

The eye pad is an oval gauze dressing that is applied over the patient's closed eyelid after ophthalmic surgery (see Fig. 2-23). The purpose of this dressing is threefold: to keep the eyelid closed to allow the eye to rest, to absorb any drainage from the eye, and to keeping medications from seeping out of the eye.

The eye shield is a rigid raised oval shield that is placed over the eye or eye dressing. The purpose of the shield is to protect the eye from trauma or pressure postoperatively. The shield can be made of rigid plastic or metal. The edge of the oval that rests on the patient's face is covered with a soft material to prevent skin damage.

Occlusive Dressings

Occlusive dressings are made of a fine mesh material that has been impregnated with a petroleum-based substance (e.g., Vaseline) to provide an airtight and watertight seal. The two most common types of occlusive dressing are Vaseline gauze and Xeroform gauze (see Fig. 2-24).

The petroleum-based substance on the dressing prevents it from sticking to the wound while the mesh allows drainage to seep into the absorbent gauze dressing placed over it. This type of dressing is often used over a suture line to protect it and to keep the absorbent gauze dressing layers from sticking to it. It also can be used around a chest tube insertion site to prevent outside air from entering the chest around the stab wound site.

Vaseline dressings are available in sheets or rolls. Sizes range from 1 × 8 inches to 6 × 36 inches. The most common sizes of Xeroform dressings are 1 × 8 inches and 5 × 9 inches.

Adaptic

Adaptic is gauze that has been impregnated with a petroleum-based substance. Unlike the Vaseline or Xeroform dressing, Adaptic is nonocclusive. It does *not* provide a watertight or airtight seal. Adaptic does, however, provide a nonadhering layer that wicks drainage away from the wound and allows the dressing to be removed without sticking (see Fig. 2-25). Adaptic is available in three sizes: 3 × 3 inches, 3 × 8 inches and 3 × 16 inches.

Telfa

Telfa is a nonadhering dressing material. It is made of absorbent gauze that is bonded on both sides with a nonadherent material to prevent it from sticking to the wound. It allows air to reach the wound and wicks the drainage away from the wound (see Fig. 2-26). Telfa is available in three sizes: 2 × 3 inches, 3 × 4 inches and 6 × 10 inches.

Telfa also can be used as a mat for tissue specimens. The nonadherent covering keeps the specimen from sticking, thus preserving the tissue integrity. Scrubbed personnel often place small tissue specimens on a piece of Telfa to keep them from becoming lost.

Tegaderm

Tegaderm is a thin, transparent, waterproof film dressing. It is used as an outer dressing for wounds from which large amounts of drainage are not expected or as a stand alone dressing over intravenous (IV) sites. One advantage of Tegaderm is that it is clear, allowing visualization of the dressing or IV site underneath it (see Fig. 2-27). Tegaderm is available in sizes ranging from 2¾ × 2¾ inches to 8 × 12 inches.

FIGURE 2-23 Eye pad and eye shield.

FIGURE 2-25 Adaptic.

FIGURE 2-24 Vaseline and Xeroform gauzes.

FIGURE 2-26 Telfa.

Island dressings

Island dressings combine a nonadherent gauze dressing with a nonirritating adhesive border. The built-in adhesive border allows these dressings to adhere directly to the skin, negating the need to use tape or a wrap to secure them (see Fig. 2-28). These dressings are used on wounds from which large amounts of drainage are not expected. Two of the most common brand names are Covaderm and Primapore. These dressings come in a variety of shapes (e.g., square, round and rectangular) and sizes.

Dressing Wraps

WATCH OUT!	**Wrapping Bandages**

Use caution when wrapping any bandage (regardless of material) in a circular fashion that encompasses the entire diameter of an extremity or other body part. The bandage should fit snugly so that it does not slide off but it should NOT be wrapped so tight that it causes circulatory problems.

After wrapping the bandage, check the areas distal to the bandage for signs of impaired circulation: cyanosis, skin coolness, skin mottling or patient complaints of numbness or tingling.

Kerlix

Kerlix (see Fig. 2-29) is a six-ply roll of loosely woven gauze material. Generally used to secure a dressing or splint in place, it conforms to the contours of the patient's body, allowing freedom of movement. It also can be used to help apply pressure to a wound or to pack a large wound.

Kerlix is available as a 4½-inch × 4-yard or 2¼-inch × 3-yard roll. Kerlix is also available as a dressing sponge impregnated with an antimicrobial substance.

Kling

Kling (see Fig. 2-29) is a roll of nonwoven gauze material used to secure bandages or splints or to provide pressure to a wound. It conforms to body contours, allowing freedom of movement. It is available in 1-, 2-, 3-, 4- or 6-inch widths.

Ace Bandage

An Ace bandage (also known as an *Ace wrap*) is a roll of elastic bandage commonly used to provide support to a sprain or strain of a joint (see Fig. 2-30). It also can be used to secure a dressing or to hold a splint in place.

FIGURE 2-27 Tegaderm.

FIGURE 2-29 Kerlix and Kling.

FIGURE 2-28 Island dressings.

FIGURE 2-30 Ace wrap.

FIGURE 2–31 Coban (Self-adherent wraps).

The elastic in the bandage allows it to stretch to conform to the area and provide limited freedom of movement. Ace bandages can be secured with tape, although most come with metal fasteners or Velcro closures. Available sizes are 2-, 3-, 4- and 6-inch widths.

Self-Adherent Wraps

Self-adherent wraps are made of a blend of nonwoven fibers and elastic to allow for stretch. They contain a cohesive material designed to allow the bandage to stick to itself but not to skin or other materials (see Fig. 2-31). These bandages are used to secure dressings or splints in place. The two most common brand names for this type of dressing are Coban and Flex-wrap. Self-adherent wraps are available in widths ranging from 1 to 6 inches.

Packings

As the name implies, packing materials are packed inside the wound to provide support, to provide hemostasis or to allow wound drainage and healing (see Fig. 2-32). Uses include boils, abscesses, fistulas and other draining or tunneling wounds as well as packing nasal passages, the rectum and the vagina.

Packings are usually made of a long strip of gauze material that is plain or impregnated with antimicrobial substances such as iodoform or silver. Creams (e.g., estrogen cream or hemorrhoid cream) may be used to coat plain packing for use after specific types of surgery.

Packing material is available in widths ranging from ¼ inch to 4 inches.

Liquid Chemical Dressings

Collodion

Collodion is a thick, yellow liquid consisting of pyroxylin mixed with alcohol and ether (see Fig. 2-33). As the solvent evaporates, collodion dries to form a waterproof film over the wound. This type of dressing is used on small wounds from which drainage is not expected. It is highly flammable and has a strong odor.

Collodion is applied over the dry suture or staple line using a cotton-tipped applicator. A thin layer is applied and left open to the air to dry. Once dry, the film provides protection from environmental contaminants and water.

Liquid Skin Adhesives

This category of dressings consists of topically applied liquid adhesives that are designed to close small, superficial lacerations and surgical incisions. In addition to wound closure they provide a chemical film barrier for protection. Brand names include Dermabond, New-Skin and LiquiBand. These adhesives come in small ampules with an applicator on one end (see Fig. 2-34). The ampule is squeezed, allowing the adhesive to saturate the applicator. A thin layer of adhesive is applied to the wound and allowed to dry and then another layer is applied (application techniques may vary with brand; always follow the manufacturer's instructions).

Prior to use, it is important to check patient allergies to make sure it is appropriate to use these adhesives (e.g., Dermabond contains formaldehyde and cannot be used on patients with formaldehyde allergies).

FIGURE 2–32 Plain and iodoform packing strip.

FIGURE 2–33 Collodion.

FIGURE 2–34 Dermabond.

Adhesive Tapes

Medical adhesive tape (also known as *surgical tape*) is the most common method of securing dressings. Available in many types and widths, it is an easy and inexpensive way to keep dressings in place. Listed are the most common types of adhesive tape:

- *Paper tape:* Hypoallergenic. Leaves very little adhesive residue when removed and is gentle on the skin. Used on patients with adhesive sensitivities or patients who have friable (fragile) skin. Good for use when repeated dressing changes are anticipated on sensitive skin. Used by some anesthesia personnel to tape eyelids shut during general anesthesia. Tends not to stick well when wet. Available in ½-, 1-, 2- and 3-inch widths. Common brand names include Micropore, Hypo-Pore and Tenderskin.
- *Silk tape:* "Silk-like tape." Most commonly used general purpose adhesive tape (see Fig. 2-35). Hypoallergenic adhesive leaves tape residue after removal. Available in ½-, 1-, 2- and 3-inch widths. Common brand names include Durapore and Hypo Silk.
- *Elastic tape:* Cotton elastic tape (see Fig. 2-36) designed for use for pressure dressings or support strapping of orthopedic injuries. Conforms to knees, shoulders and elbows. Allows for wicking of moisture away from the skin. Has a rubber-based adhesive. Available in 1-, 2-, 3- and 4-inch widths. Common brand names include Elastoplast and Elastikon.
- *Plastic tape:* Flexible, contouring, clear plastic tape that allows viewing of the wound site. Used for securing dressings, IV catheters or tubes. Available in 1-, 2- or 3-inch widths. Brand names include Blenderm, Transpore, DermiView and HypoClear.
- *Fabric tape:* Porous and nonabsorbing fabric used to secure dressings, tubes and cannulas. Nonirritating adhesive allows skin underneath it to breath. Available in

1-, 2-, 4-, 6- and 8-inch widths; brand names include Hypafix and Mefix.
- *Foam elastic tape:* Elastic foam material (see Fig. 2-36) used for compression dressing or dressing in hard-to-secure areas. Stretches in all directions. Waterproof and hypoallergenic. Available in 1-, 2-, 3- and 4-inch widths. Common brand name is Microfoam.
- *Cloth tape:* Nonwoven polyester tape (see Fig. 2-35). Easy to tear, hypoallergenic, general purpose tape. Has moderate stretch to allow for movement and swelling. Available in 1-, 2-, 3-, 4-, 6- and 8-inch widths. Brand names include Dermicel and Curasilk.
- *Waterproof tape:* Zinc oxide–based tape (see Fig. 2-35). Waterproof and oil resistant and gentle to all skin types, it will remain intact for long periods of time, even when wet. Conforms easily to body contours. Used to secure dressings or tubes. Used by some anesthesia personnel to secure endotracheal tubes. Available in ½-, 1-, and 2-inch widths. Brand names include Hy-Tape, Scanpor, Wet Pruf and Megazinc.

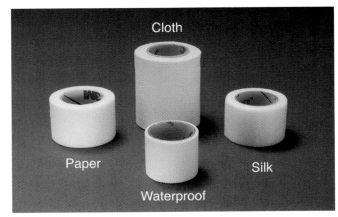

FIGURE 2–35 Paper, silk, cloth and waterproof tapes.

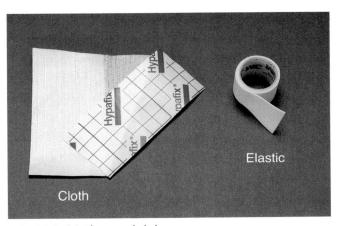

FIGURE 2–36 Elastic and cloth tapes.

Casting Material (Rigid Dressings)

Plaster

Plaster bandages are made from cotton material that is impregnated with plaster of Paris. To apply, the material is dipped in water and wrapped in place. The plaster hardens as it dries, creating a hard shell that provides support and protection to the surgical or fracture site. Plaster casting material is both strong and easy to manipulate, making it a popular choice for creating casts. The disadvantage to plaster is that it becomes mushy and looses it shape and supporting ability when it becomes wet. It is also heavier than fiberglass, making it uncomfortable for some patients.

Plaster casting material is available in rolls (for applying casts) or strips (for making splints) ranging from 2 to 6 inches wide (see Fig. 2-37).

Fiberglass

Fiberglass casting material has become popular because it is lightweight and holds it shape better than plaster when it is exposed to moisture. These bandages consist of a knitted fiberglass bandage impregnated with polyurethane. To apply, the fiberglass material is dipped in water and wrapped it place. As it dries, it forms a protective and supportive shell around the surgical or fracture site. Fiberglass dries quicker than plaster and, as it hardens, the chemical reaction causes the casting material to become warm. It is a good idea to tell the patient that as the cast dries, it will feel warm.

Fiberglass casting material is available in rolls (for applying casts) or pre-cut (for making splints) of various sizes and widths (see Fig. 2-37).

Webril

Webril is a soft cotton padding material applied to the skin before a cast or pneumatic tourniquet is fitted. Webril provides protection and padding (see Fig. 2-38). It is soft, contours to the body and stays in place without shifting or sagging. Webril is not waterproof; therefore, if the patient gets the cast wet, the Webril could absorb some of the water and hold it next to the skin, causing skin irritation or breakdown.

FIGURE 2-38 Webril.

Webril is available in rolls ranging from 2 to 6 inch widths.

Stockinette

Stockinette is available in several styles that can be used to pad under casting material (to prevent chafing), to drape an extremity for surgery or to hold a dressing in place. It also can be placed over a device such as a cervical collar to help keep it clean. When the stockinette becomes soiled, slip it off and either wash it or apply a new one.

As the name implies, stockinette is a round tube of soft cotton material that is applied by slipping it onto the extremity or torso like you would put on a stocking (see Fig. 2-39). It is stretchy, lightweight and breathable. Stockinette comes in a tubular roll and is available in widths ranging from 1 to 12 inches.

Miscellaneous

Skin Closure Tapes

Commonly referred to by the brand name *Steri-Strips* (3M company), skin closure tapes are polyester-reinforced strips of material with a hypoallergenic adhesive backing (see Fig. 2-40). They can be used to close a wound or incision or to reinforce a sutured incision line. The most commonly used sizes are ¼- and ½-inch wide.

FIGURE 2-37 Plaster and fiberglass casting materials.

Fiberglass

Plaster

Impervious

Regular

Loosely woven

FIGURE 2-39 Regular, impervious and loosely woven stockinettes.

FIGURE 2-40 Steri-Strips.

FIGURE 2-42 Mastisol.

Tincture of Benzoin

This is an alcohol compound containing benzoin that can be used to help increase the adhesion of Steri-Strips or dressings. Once it is dry it forms a protective film on the skin. Available in swabs or ⅔-mL ampules (see Fig. 2-41).

Mastisol

Mastisol is a clear, nonirritating, non–water-soluble adhesive that helps secure dressings for a prolonged period of time. Often, it is used in conjunction with Tegaderm dressings. Mastisol is 7 to 10 times stickier than benzoin. Available in ⅔-mL ampules and 15-mL and 60-mL bottles (see Fig. 2-42).

Montgomery Straps

Montgomery straps are large adhesive strips that are placed opposite each other. The straps have holes along the inner edge to allow them to be threaded with gauze or twill tape to secure the dressing (see Fig. 2-43).

The advantage to Montgomery straps is that the dressing can be accessed and changed without having to change the adhesive. Generally, these are used for large wounds for which frequent dressing changes are expected. Available in 7¼- × 11⅛-inch sizes, they can be cut to the desired length.

FIGURE 2-43 Montgomery straps.

Ostomy Appliances

Ostomy appliances (also known as *stoma bags* or *ostomy bags*) are available in many sizes and styles depending on the desired use and patient preference. These appliances have an opening near the top where the ostomy effluent drains into the bag and many have a re-closable opening at the bottom of the bag to allow for emptying. The bags may be one piece where the adhesive seal that goes around the stoma is built into the bag (see Fig. 2-44A) or two piece where the adhesive seal is separate and the bag attaches to it (see Fig. 2-44B). The adhesive seal is circular; on some styles it can be cut to fit the stoma and some models it is a fixed size. The most common ostomy appliances are used for patients with urostomies, ileostomies and colostomies.

Many institutions employ an ostomy nurse who is responsible for helping patients preoperatively and postoperatively with fitting of appliance, caring for the stoma, and learning to live/cope with an ostomy. These nurses are a valuable resource for the perioperative team.

Vacuum-Assisted Closure Dressings

Vacuum-assisted closure (VAC) dressings are designed to apply negative pressure to chronic wounds to help accelerate the

FIGURE 2-41 Benzoin.

FIGURE 2–44 A) One-piece and B) two-piece ostomy bags.

healing process. Examples of wounds that VAC dressings can be used for include chronic ulcers, skin grafts, flaps, traumatic wounds and partial-thickness burns.

There are two parts to the VAC dressing: the vacuum machine and the foam sponge dressing. The foam sponge is placed into the open wound, the wound is sealed with an adhesive drape and the sponge's hose is attached to the vacuum machine's hose (see Fig. 2-45). Negative pressure is then applied to the wound using the machine.

VAC dressing sponges are available in two different foam materials. GranuFoam is designed to remove exudate and assist in wound granulation. Vers-Foam is a nonadherent material that helps promote graft survival, helps protect underlying structures and can be used in wounds with tunnels or undermining.

VAC foam sponges are available in various sizes to fit hands, heels and abdomen, although they can be used for wounds in other parts of the body. The vacuum machine is available in a floor model (larger size) or a small, portable model that comes

with a case that the patient can attach to a strap to carry around. For more information, see www.KCI1.com.

FIGURE 2–45 Vacuum machine and foam dressing.

Drapes

Name: x-ray cassette drape

Alias: none

Use: covers an x-ray cassette that needs to be placed in the sterile field

Features: deep cuff to protect the hands of scrub personnel

Additional Information: available in several sizes, ranging from 14 × 19 inches to 24 × 40 inches; clear plastic so that cassette can be seen easily for placement

Name: microscope drape
Alias: none
Use: drapes the microscope for use in the surgical field
Features: tape closures ensure custom fit around oculars
Additional Information: available to fit several models of microscope

Name: camera drape
Alias: camera/laser arm drape
Use: drapes a nonsterile camera or a laser arm for use in the surgical field
Features: clear plastic so that equipment can be seen easily; telescopically folded for ease of application
Additional Information: 96 inches long; end width available in 5 or 7 inches

Name: C-arm drape
Alias: x-ray image intensifier drape
Use: drapes C-arm for use in the sterile field
Features: one-piece coverage; adhesive strips or patches help to customize fit to machine
Additional Information: available in sizes to fit regular C-arm or mini C-arm models

Name: banded bag
Alias: bonnet
Use: covers equipment that is going to be used in the sterile field; some surgeons use it to cover the end of the C-arm
Features: clear plastic to allow for equipment visualization; nonlatex elastic opening
Additional Information: available with 17-, 23-, 35- or 45-inch opening

Name: ultrasound probe drape

Alias: none

Use: drapes probes for use in the sterile field

Features: available with several tips to accommodate different styles of probes (e.g., straight tip, angled tip, T-tip and burr hole tip)

Additional Information: 5 × 96 inches; telescopically folded for ease of application

Name: incise drape

Alias: none

Use: creates a sterile operative area up to the wound edges

Features: provides a barrier to skin bacteria

Additional Information: available in many sizes ranging from 4 × 8 inches to 23 × 33 inches; latex-free

Name: Ioban

Alias: antimicrobial incise drape

Use: provides a sterile surface up to the wound edges; provides continuous anti-microbial activity intraoperatively

Features: stretches and contours to accommodate surgical site manipulation

Additional Information: available in several sizes ranging from 4 × 8 inches to 23 × 33 inches; latex free; cannot be used on patients with iodine sensitivity or allergy

Name: impervious stockinette

Alias: none

Use: drapes extremity

Features: fluid-proof barrier helps to reduce the chance of microbial migration

Additional Information: available in 8-, 10- or 12-inch widths; some available with straps to help ease over the extremity

Impervious stockinette

Name: impervious split drape

Alias: none

Use: drapes the top of an extremity (e.g., drapes the top of the thigh/buttock for hip surgery)

Features: split makes it easy to wrap around the extremity; fluid-proof

Additional Information: 60 × 70 inches; large size is 60 × 81 inches; available with or without a built-in pouch

Name: extremity drape
Alias: none
Use: drapes an arm or leg
Features: 2.5-inch stretchable circular fenestration
Additional Information: 90 × 124 inches
Name: lower extremity drape
Alias: lower limb drape
Use: drapes the leg
Features: 2.5-inch stretchable circular fenestration
Additional Information: 88 × 122 inches

Name: bilateral limb drape
Alias: bilateral extremity drape
Use: drapes both legs at the same time (e.g., draping for bilateral knee arthroplasties)
Features: two 2.5-inch stretchable circular fenestrations
Additional Information: 76 × 120 inches

Name: beach chair shoulder drape
Alias: none
Use: drapes out the shoulder for open shoulder procedures
Features: available with or without a pouch
Additional Information: 172 × 100 inches

Name: laparotomy drape
Alias: none
Use: draping the abdomen for general or gynecological surgery
Features: 4 × 12 inch fenestration; attached arm board covers; attached tube holders
Additional Information: available in several adult and pediatric sizes; fenestration can be vertical (for midline incisions) or horizontal

Name: laparoscopic cholecystectomy drape
Alias: lap chole drape
Use: drapes the abdomen for laparoscopic cholecystectomy
Features: 12 × 13.5 inch laterally offset fenestration
Additional Information: 104 × 120 inches; available with or without instrument pouch

Name: cesarean section drape
Alias: C-section drape
Use: drapes the abdomen for a cesarean section
Features: fenestrated incise area with large 360-degree fluid collection pouch
Additional Information: 100 × 72 × 120 inches

Name: under buttocks drape
Alias: none
Use: drape placed under the buttocks for gynecological procedures
Features: fluid-proof
Additional Information: available in small, medium and large sizes

Name: utility drape
Alias: towel drape
Use: squares off the incision area
Features: built-in adhesive strip holds the drape in place
Additional Information: 15 × 26 inches; comes in a package of two; some surgeons use these in place of linen towels

Name: half drape

Alias: none

Use: general purpose drape (e.g., can be used to drape arm boards and x-ray cassettes and cover small utility table)

Features: comes one to a package; able to be folded to fit the area needed; has no adhesive; may need to use towel clamp to hold it in place

Additional Information: 60 × 44 inches

Name: large drape

Alias: none

Use: used as general purpose drape to cover large areas

Features: comes one to a package; no adhesive

Additional Information: 60 × 76 inches

Name: back table cover

Alias: none

Use: drapes instrument or table (back tables)

Features: reinforced for extra tear resistance; impervious backing to prevent fluid strike through

Additional Information: 44 × 90 inches

Name: overhead table cover

Alias: none

Use: drapes Mayfield (overhead) table

Features: sterile skirt around drape extends the sterile field to the top surface of the draped patient

Additional Information: available in regular or extra large sizes

Name: leggings

Alias: none

Use: drape the feet and legs of patients who are in stirrups

Features: some drapes have clear tops so that feet and legs can be seen; drapes are marked "right" and "left"

Additional Information: come as a pair; have cuff to protect scrub person's hands while applying the drape

Name: U-bar drape

Alias: bar drape

Use: usually used to drape chest or abdomen

Features: drape with a U cut out; 4 × 40-inch split (chest drape has 12 × 30-inch split)

Additional Information: 76 × 120 inches

Name: arthroscopy drape

Alias: none

Use: drapes extremity for arthroscopic surgery

Features: 2.5-inch stretchable circular fenestration; fluid collection pouch with suction port

Additional Information: 90 × 124 inches

Name: cystoscopy drape

Alias: none

Use: drapes perineal area and abdomen for cysto-scopic procedures

Features: T shape allows coverage of legs and abdomen with narrow part draping the perineum; 3 × 6-inch fenestration allows access to the perineal area

Additional Information: available in two sizes

Name: Mayo stand cover

Alias: none

Use: drapes standard size Mayo stand

Features: reinforced to help prevent tears; impervious backing helps prevent strike through contamination

Additional Information: 23 × 54 inches

Name: extra-large Mayo stand cover

Alias: none

Use: drapes large Mayo stands

Features: reinforced to help prevent tears; impervious backing helps prevent strike through contamination

Additional Information: 30 × 57 inches; large Mayo stands are often used in orthopedic, neurosurgery or spine cases

Name: head drape

Alias: turban drape

Use: drapes the head and covers the hair for eye, ear, nose and throat (EENT) surgery

Features: has built-in turban to cover the patient's hair and keep it out of the operative field

Additional Information: available in two sizes (36 × 24 inches and 33 × 20 inches)

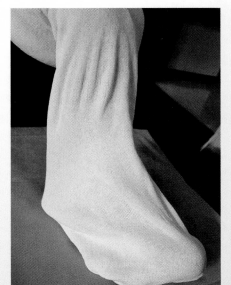

Name: stockinette

Alias: none

Use: drapes an extremity

Features: not impervious; comes in 3- to 6-ft rolls to make it easier to apply to the extremity

Additional Information: available in 2-, 4-, 6- or 8-inch widths

Name: craniotomy drape

Alias: none

Use: drapes the patient's head and body during a craniotomy

Features: oval fenestration; clear panels to allow anesthesia to visualize the patient

Additional Information: 122 × 74 × 134 inches

Name: EENT drape

Alias: none

Use: drapes the patient's head and body for EENT procedures

Features: available in two styles: one with a 3 × 28-inch split and one with a 2 × 2.5-inch fenestration

Additional Information: split drape is 76 × 124 inches; fenestrated drape is 76 × 90 inches

Name: ophthalmic drape

Alias: eye drape

Use: drapes the patient's eye, head and upper body during ophthalmic procedures

Features: 3 × 2-inch oval fenestration; fluid collection pouch

Additional Information: 52 × 56 inches

Name: woven towel

Alias: woven towel; cloth towel

Use: drapes the surgical site; covers Mayo stand or portions of the back table; can be rolled to make a place to hold instruments

Features: washable and sterilizable; generally packaged four or eight to a pack; if used to drape the surgical site either towel clips or incise/loban drapes can be used to hold them in place

Additional Information: Be cautious when using sharps so as not to slice the drape; it is <u>not</u> impervious to fluids

Name: incise utility towel
Alias: none
Use: drapes the surgical field (used like woven towel or utility drape)
Features: adhesive strip holds it in place; clear, which allows visualization around the wound area
Additional Information: none

Name: woven sheet
Alias: cloth sheet
Use: generally covers a back table cover to give extra reinforcement; can be used as a sterile drape for the patient (e.g., could be put on a stretcher where a burn patient is going to be placed or used to cover a burn patient)
Features: washable and sterilizable
Additional Information: not impervious to fluids

Name: breast/chest drape
Alias: none
Use: drapes patient for breast or thoracic procedures
Features: 13 × 14-inch fenestration; arm board covers; instrument pad
Additional Information: 100 × 72 × 124 inches

Name: CV drape
Alias: cardiovascular drape
Use: drapes the body, leaving the leg exposed for cardiovascular surgery (e.g., for femoral-popliteal bypass surgery or for harvesting of leg vein for cardiac bypasses)
Features: split all the way down allowing one leg to be completely exposed; tubing pockets
Additional Information: 116 × 88 × 140 inches; 92-inch long split

Name: split body drape
Alias: none
Use: used as general purpose split body drape for orthopedic surgery
Features: 27-inch split
Additional Information: 88 × 116 inches

Name: controller drape
Alias: none
Use: drapes equipment remote controls
Features: drape is opened like a plastic bag and the nonsterile remote is dropped inside
Additional Information: none

SKIN PREPPING SOLUTIONS

The most common cause of surgical site infection is the normal bacteria (flora) found on the skin of the patient or surgical team members. In order to decrease the number of bacteria found on the patient's skin to an absolute minimum, the skin is prepped at the surgical site before the patient is draped. The prep removes oil and dirt that can harbor harmful bacteria and minimizes the normal bacteria on the skin.

Several solutions can be used to prepare the patient's skin before surgery. The type of prepping solution used depends on the area to be prepped and the patient's allergy history. The only solutions that are used as prep agents are those that are approved for use on the skin. Use of any other type of agents (e.g., disinfectants or chemical sterilants) could result in severe damage to the patient's skin. Covered in this section are the four most commonly used prepping solutions: alcohol, iodophors (povidone-iodine), DuraPrep and chlorhexidine gluconate.

Alcohol

The most common alcohol solutions used for skin preparation are those containing 70% isopropyl alcohol. At this concentration, the solution is 95% effective against both gram-positive and gram-negative bacteria; however, it is not completely effective against their spores. Alcohol works to kill bacteria by drying out the cell proteins. It is this drying characteristic that makes alcohol *not* appropriate for use on mucous membranes, in open wounds or in eyes.

Isopropyl alcohol is colorless, although some places add a blue color to make it easier to distinguish from saline or other clear medications and solutions. It has a strong odor and is highly flammable. This flammability makes it imperative that the skin be given *adequate time to dry* prior to applying drapes; *all* traces of the alcohol must be gone. If alcohol is still present on the skin or drapes when laser or electrocautery is used, a fire could result.

Isopropyl alcohol in a 70% solution is available on swabs, on pads, in bottles or in spray bottles. The most common container

seen in the OR for skin prep is the 16-oz bottle (see Fig. 2-46). Isopropyl alcohol is also available in a 99% solution (bottle and spray bottle), although this is not as commonly used.

Iodophors

Iodophors are a combination of iodine and povidone, which helps to make the iodine less irritating to tissue. The common concentration of povidone-iodine solution used for surgical skin prep is 10%. This type of solution is often referred to by the brand name *Betadine*.

In addition to the solution (sometimes referred to in the OR as *paint*), iodophors are mixed with detergents to make a 7.5% "scrub" solution. The scrub solution can be used by personnel to scrub their hands and arms before entering the sterile field or can be used to wash the patient's skin before applying the paint solution. Unlike the solution (or paint), iodophor scrub is *not* meant to be left on the skin and must be rinsed off. Scrub solutions should *not* be used around the eyes or on mucous membranes, although the paint solution can be used in these areas.

FIGURE 2–46 Isopropyl alcohol.

Iodophors are effective against gram-positive bacteria, but they are not as effective against gram-negative bacteria, viruses and fungi. They do provide some residual antimicrobial effect.

Iodophor solution is available in bottles, on swab sticks, on pads and in spray bottles (see Fig. 2-47). The scrub solution is available in bottles and on surgical scrub brushes. Due to the iodine content in this product, it *should not* be used on patients with an iodine allergy.

DuraPrep

DuraPrep is the 3M brand name for a popular prepping solution that combines 70% isopropyl alcohol and iodophor solution. The combination of the solutions combines the fast bacterial killing action of alcohol with the residual effect of the iodophor (kills bacteria up to 12 hours). It contains alcohol; therefore, it is flammable and must be allowed to dry completely (about 3 minutes) before applying drapes.

DuraPrep is packaged in a self-contained sponge applicator for ease of prep (see Fig. 2-48). The applicator is available in two sizes: 6 mL (for small areas) and 26 mL (for larger areas).

Once applied, DuraPrep forms an antimicrobial film that can be difficult to remove. DuraPrep can be removed from the skin postoperatively using DuraPrep Remover.

Chlorhexidine Gluconate

Chlorhexidine gluconate is used as in a 4% solution for surgical skin prep or as a surgical hand scrub (see Fig. 2-49). Upon application, it has a broad-spectrum antimicrobial effect and has a residual effect of up to 5 to 6 hours. One of the more common brand names for this solution is Hibiclens.

For surgical skin preparation, the manufacturer suggests chlorhexidine gluconate solution be applied to the skin and swabbed around for 2 minutes. The area is then dried with a sterile towel, and the solution is reapplied and swabbed for 2 more minutes. The area is then dried again with a sterile towel. (Skin preparation procedures vary among institutions; check your institution's policy or procedure.)

Chlorhexidine gluconate has been associated with hearing loss when introduced into the middle ear; therefore, it should *never be used* for preparations around the ear. It also *should not* be used for preparation of the eye, of the mouth or on large open wounds.

This solution is available in bottles of varying sizes and on surgical scrub brushes.

FIGURE 2–48 DuraPrep.

FIGURE 2–47 Iodophor solution and scrub bottles.

FIGURE 2–49 Chlorhexidine gluconate.

BASINS

Name: graduate

Alias: none

Use: holds and measures irrigation fluids

Features: marked in cubic centimeters (cc) to allow fluid measurement; most common size is 1000 cc

Additional Information: available in metal or plastic versions; all fluids, solutions and medications on the sterile field should be labeled

Name: alcohol cup

Alias: paint cup

Use: holds prep solution or medication

Features: able to fit in one hand so that it can be held by the person painting the skin (prep)

Additional Information: all fluids, solutions and medications on the sterile field should be labeled

Name: medication cup

Alias: none

Use: holds and measures medications and solutions

Features: marked in cubic centimeters (cc) to allow for ease of measurement

Additional Information: available in plastic or metal versions; most common size holds 2 oz (60 cc); all fluids, solutions and medications on the sterile field should be labeled

Name: round bowl

Alias: none

Use: stores solutions or medication on the back table; contains the specimen before it is passed off to the circulator

Features: available in many sizes to accommodate various uses

Additional Information: available in stainless steel or plastic disposal styles

Name: wash bowl

Alias: extra large basin

Use: soaks instruments intraoperatively; contains large specimens before passing them to the circulator; in some institutions, wash bowls are used to open small items into when first opening the supplies

Features: large capacity

Additional Information: available in stainless steel or plastic disposable styles

Name: soaking basin

Alias: none

Use: soaks instruments intraoperatively

Features: large capacity; rectangular shape allows for soaking of long instruments (e.g., femoral reamers)

Additional Information: available in shallow or deep styles

OTHER SUPPLIES

Name: suture boots

Alias: shods

Use: protect sutures from damage that serrated instrument jaws can cause

Features: soft plastic; fit onto the tips of mosquitos (Halstead) or Crile clamps

Additional Information: come in packages of 10; may be included as part of the count

Name: clamp cover
Alias: pants
Use: covers the blades of Doyen clamps to protect delicate tissue
Features: available in wide or narrow
Additional Information: dipping into saline before applying to the clamp blade makes it easier to put on and makes it wet and ready to use; may be included as part of the count

Name: vessel loops
Alias: none
Use: retract vessels during surgery
Features: available in red (arteries) or blue (veins)
Additional Information: available in narrow or wide; may be included as part of the count

Name: umbilical tape
Alias: cotton tape
Use: ties off umbilical cord; retracts or ties vessels
Features: soft, nontraumatic to vessels or tissue
Additional Information: may be included as part of the count; should be moistened with saline before use

Name: Raney clips
Alias: scalp clips
Use: retracts scalp tissue out of the way during cranial surgery
Features: plastic; single patient use
Additional Information: need to be loaded onto a manual applier for use

Name: medication labels
Alias: none
Use: labels medication and solution containers on the field
Features: may be blank or pre-printed
Additional Information: self-stick backing allows for application directly to the containers

Name: umbilical cord clamp

Alias: cord clamp

Use: clamps off the umbilical cord after birth

Features: clamp tip facilitates easy closure and secure hold

Additional Information: single patient use; have open on Mayo stand prior to delivery during a C-section

Name: ruler

Alias: none

Use: measures wounds, grafts, implants and so on

Features: markings in inches and centimeters

Additional Information: available in paper (single patient use) or metal (re-sterilizable)

Name: surgical marker

Alias: marking pen

Use: marks the skin

Features: available with a medium or fine point; some have rulers marked on the side

Additional Information: single patient use

Name: winged infusion set

Alias: port access needle; Huber needle

Use: accesses implanted ports for infusion of fluids or medication

Features: noncoring so that it will not damage the port

Additional Information: available in a variety of gauge sizes; single patient use

Name: defogger kit

Alias: none

Use: defogs camera and scope lenses

Features: comes with liquid and sponge applicator

Additional Information: single patient use

Name: decanting cannula

Alias: none

Use: pours fluid from a sterile IV bag to a container on the sterile field

Features: has a spiked end to insert into the port on the bottom of the bag

Additional Information: care must be taken not to contaminate the tip while pouring

Name: Hydrajaw insert

Alias: Fogarty insert

Use: pads the jaws of Fogarty clamps to minimize tissue damage

Features: has clips on the inner side to attach to the clamp jaws; outer side padded

Additional Information: none

Name: remover lotion

Alias: DuraPrep Remover

Use: removes excess DuraPrep solution from the skin after surgery

Features: easy to apply; just rub onto skin

Additional Information: rub onto skin and remove with a dry, clean towel or sponge

Name: water soluble jelly

Alias: K-Y Jelly; Surgilube

Use: lubricates tubes and catheters before insertion into body orifices

Features: water soluble; easy to clean off excess

Additional Information: comes sterile in a variety of containers (from small packets to large tubes); spike on cap is used to puncture tube seal

Name: povidone-iodine swab

Alias: Betadine swab

Use: cleansing small areas of skin

Features: swab impregnated with povidone-iodine, thus eliminating the need for a separate container of solution

Additional Information: available in packages of one to three swabs

Name: magnetic drape

Alias: none

Use: keeps metal instruments from slipping off the draped patient and onto the floor

Features: rows of magnets that keep metal instruments from slipping off

Additional Information: available in a variety of styles and sizes

Name: culture tube

Alias: Culturette

Use: obtains and contains fluid sample to send for culture

Features: sterile swab is used to obtain culture then placed in the tube with culture media in it

Additional Information: swab and inside of media tube are sterile; care must be taken not to contaminate either when placing the swab back into the tube.

Name: Whitacre spinal needle

Alias: none

Use: creates a pathway for the introduction of regional anesthetics into the spinal canal for spinal analgesia and anesthesia; can be used to inject medication into deep or hard to reach areas (e.g., the cervix)

Features: pencil point tip; 3.5 to 5.5 inches long

Additional Information: available in 18-gauge to 27-gauge sizes; available in regular or high-flow style

Name: specimen containers

Alias: none

Use: contain and preserve tissue specimens being sent to the laboratory

Features: some containers are prefilled with preservative (left photograph); some containers do not contain any preservative and can be used for frozen section specimens as well; if you are sending a specimen that requires a preservative in a dry container, preservative must be added and the container properly labeled (right photograph)

Additional Information: both styles come in a variety of sizes to accommodate most specimens

Name: Jamshidi needle

Alias: bone marrow needle

Use: injects fluid or medication into the bone marrow (intraosseous infusion); aspirates bone marrow for biopsy; harvests bone graft from the iliac crest

Features:

Additional Information: available in several gauges (8 gauge to 17 gauge); available in several lengths

Name: Tru-cut biopsy needle

Alias: none

Use: obtains tissue samples from organs for examination

Features:

Additional Information: available in several gauges (14 gauge to 27 gauge); available in 3-, 4.5- and 6-inch lengths

Name: specimen cup

Alias: urine cup

Use: sends specimens to the laboratory that should not have a preservative or fluid with them (e.g., renal stones, frozen sections); collects a urine specimen

Features: inside of cup is sterile

Additional Information: these containers could be used for any specimen, but if a preservative (e.g., formalin) is required, the preservative must be added and the proper label affixed to the container; available in many sizes

Name: sputum trap

Alias: none

Use: collects sputum specimen

Features: attaches to suction to allow for collecting the specimen directly by using suction to draw it into the container

Additional Information: marked in cubic centimeters to allow for estimating specimen volume

Name: urine strainer

Alias: none

Use: strains urine specimen to check for the presence of stones, gravel or tissue

Features: end is Micro-Mesh to allow urine to filter through but to capture any stones or sediment

Additional Information: many styles and types available

Name: biohazard bag

Alias: specimen bag

Use: place specimen container into it before sending to the laboratory; protects personnel if leakage occurs

Features: resealable; leak-proof if sealed properly; marked with biohazard symbol

Additional Information: available in a variety of sizes

Name: tongue blade

Alias: tongue depressor

Use: holds tongue, allowing visualization of mouth and pharynx; stirs medication mixtures

Features: comes packaged as sterile or unsterile

Additional Information: none

Name: cotton tip applicator

Alias: cotton swab

Use: applies medication to small areas; dabs blood or fluid from small areas

Features: comes packaged as sterile or unsterile

Additional Information: available in several lengths and sizes

Name: isolation bag

Alias: none

Use: isolates a body part (e.g., foot or bowel) away from the operative area

Features: sterile bag with a drawstring closure

Additional Information: if using the bag to isolate an organ such as the bowel, add sterile saline to the bag to keep the organ moist while it is outside the body

Name: Glassman viscera retainer

Alias: fish

Use: protects the viscera while suturing

Features: the body portion is inserted between the viscera and the peritoneum; when the wound is almost closed, the retainer is removed by pulling on the tail portion

Additional Information: single use

Name: Lone Star retractor

Alias: none

Use: retracts soft tissue; used mostly in vaginal and rectal surgery

Features: hooks are placed on the soft tissue then attached to the retractor frame

Additional Information: available in several sizes and styles; hooks and frame come separately so you need to make sure you have both packages

Name: sterile water

Alias: none

Use: fills Pleur-Evacs, blanket rolls or other medical equipment requiring water; soaks surgical instruments

Features: noncorrosive

Additional Information: available in several sizes; 500 cc and 1000 cc are the most common

Name: normal saline

Alias: none

Use: irrigates wounds or body cavities

Features: isotonic solution

Additional Information: corrosive to stainless steel; do not use for soaking instruments; available in several sizes; 500 cc and 1000 cc are the most common

Name: Glycine 1.5%

Alias: none

Use: irrigate body cavities during procedures requiring use of resectoscope/cautery

Features: nonconducting

Additional Information: comes in 3000-cc bag

Name: surgical nerve locator

Alias: none

Use: locates and stimulates nerves intraoperatively

Features: direct current stimulator; adjustable 0.5 mA to 2.0 mA

Additional Information: single patient use; handheld; battery powered

Name: suture bag
Alias: garbage bag
Use: use to dispose of suture wrappers, cut off pieces of suture and other waste items intraoperatively
Features: self-sticking tabs make it easier to hang on the back table
Additional Information: none

Name: handheld cautery
Alias: none
Use: cauterization of fine vessels or tissue (e.g., in hand surgery)
Features: battery powered; tip heats up
Additional Information: single patient use

Name: blade knife handle
Alias: Beaver Blade handle
Use: holds knife blades
Features: available in long or short handle lengths
Additional Information: for use with series 50, 60, 70 blades

#10 Blade: generally used for skin incisions
#11 Blade: for small "puncture" incisions (e.g., in a hook phlebectomy, arthroscopic or endoscopic procedures)
#12 Blade: curved with a cutting surface on the inside; used in oropharyngeal surgery (e.g., tonsils, uvulopalatopharyngoplasty)
#15 Blade: used for cutting small vessels and tissue, plastic surgery skin incisions and hand procedures

Name: Incontinence pad
Alias: Chux; prep pad; bed protector pad
Use: absorbs fluids; used to protect the bed linen from prep solutions or body fluids
Features: absorbent top backed by a fluid-proof backing
Additional Information: available in many sizes and styles

Name: Hypaque

Alias: diatrizoate

Use: contrast media used for intraoperative radiography

Features: clear; available in several strengths; 60% is the one most commonly used

Additional Information: make sure ALL bubbles are out of the syringe before handing it to the surgeon for injection; bubbles can resemble a stone on the x-ray image; as with all fluids and medications, make sure it is properly labeled with name and strength; use only with extreme caution in someone with an iodine sensitivity

Name: Omnipaque

Alias: Iohexol

Use: contrast media for intraoperative angiography (also used for myelography and arthrography)

Features: clear; available in several strengths (180, 240, 300 and 350); 350 is the most commonly used for intraoperative angiography

Additional Information: make sure ALL bubbles are out of the syringe before handing it to the surgeon for injection; bubbles can resemble a stone on the x-ray image; as with all fluids and medications, make sure it is properly labeled with name and strength; use only with extreme caution in someone with an iodine sensitivity

Name: polymethyl methacrylate

Alias: bone cement

Use: cements prostheses in place during total joint arthroplasty

Features: comes as a powder with one to two vials of liquid; mix only with the liquid polymer that comes with it

Additional Information: has strong vapors; excessive exposure can be potentially hazardous for staff; mix using a closed cement mixing system to decrease fumes; pregnant women should not be in the OR during the mixing of bone cement

Antibiotic bone cement   Regular bone cement

Name: polymethyl methacrylate with gentamycin

Alias: antibiotic bone cement

Use: cementing prostheses in place during total joint arthroplasty; used for patients at higher risk for infection (e.g., diabetic patients or those with a history of infection)

Features: comes as a powder with one to two vials of liquid; mix only with the liquid polymer that comes with it

Additional Information: has strong vapors; excessive exposure can be potentially hazardous for staff; mix using a closed cement mixing system to decrease fumes; pregnant women should not be in the OR during the mixing of bone cement; not for use in patients with a sensitivity to gentamycin

Name: Doppler

Alias: none

Use: assesses blood flow in arteries

Features: detachable cord so that cord can be sterile and box left unsterile; adjustable volume

Additional Information: a non-sterile probe can be used preoperatively and postoperatively, have a sterile one available intraoperatively; there are many models available

Name: Esmarch

Alias: none

Use: exsanguinates the extremity prior to surgery

Features: latex-free; comes in a roll for easy application

Additional Information: extremity is always wrapped starting at the distal point and moving toward the proximal end; available in 3-, 4- or 6-inch width; available sterile or nonsterile

Name: TUR system with flow pouch

Alias: none

Use: provides constant, high-pressure irrigation during transurethral resection procedures

Features: 2000-cc reservoir pouch; dual spikes allow two bags of irrigation fluid to be hung simultaneously

Additional Information: not latex-free

Name: Simpulse SOLO irrigator

Alias: pulsed lavage irrigator

Use: irrigating surgical sites during orthopedic procedures

Features: battery operated; no external power source needed; variable power control at located at the trigger; pistol grip

Additional Information: is a dual irrigation/ suction system

Name: sterile mineral oil

Alias: none

Use: lubricates skin prior to using a dermatome for skin grafting

Features: sterile

Additional Information: single patient use

Name: scratch pad

Alias: tip cleaner

Use: removes char and tissue from electrocautery tip

Features: adhesive backing allows it to stick to drape or holster

Additional Information: none

Name: ultrasonic gel

Alias: none

Use: provides an acoustically correct medium for the transmission of ultrasonic waves; provides lubrication for the probe to glide over the skin

Features: hypoallergenic; nonirritating to skin; non-staining

Additional Information: available in sterile packets or unsterile bottles (depending on your intended use)

 Surgical Session Review

1) Which type of sponge is <u>never</u> used as a dressing:
   a. RayTec
   b. Topper
   c. Drain sponge
   d. ABD pad

2) All of the following statements are true about sponges *except:*
   a. used sponges should be discarded off the field into a proper receptacle
   b. once initial count is done, it is OK to remove sponges from the room
   c. when setting up your back table, like sponges should be kept together
   d. never handle soiled sponges with your bare hands

3) RayTec sponges come in a package containing _____ sponges.
   a. 5
   b. 8
   c. 10
   d. 12

4) "Peanuts" may also be known as:
   a. Kitners
   b. dissectors
   c. pushers
   d. all of the above

5) Cottonoids would most likely be used during which type of surgery?
   a. gynecological
   b. neurosurgical
   c. bowel
   d. obstetrical

6) Which of the following is *not* a hemostatic?
   a. saline
   b. Avitene
   c. bone wax
   d. Collastat

7) An insulin syringe is marked in _____.
   a. cc (cubic centimeters)
   b. μg (micrograms)
   c. mg (milligrams)
   d. units

8) During which of these surgical procedures would you expect to have a blue bulb syringe on your sterile field?
   a. bowel resection
   b. cesarean section
   c. hysterectomy
   d. total hip replacement

9) Which of these needles would have the largest diameter?
   a. 16
   b. 18
   c. 25
   d. 27

10) A needle cannot be placed on the tip of a _____ syringe.
   a. Luer-lock
   b. Toomey
   c. catheter tip
   d. glass

11) _____ is a type of liquid dressing.
   a. Coban
   b. Adaptic
   c. collodion
   d. Tegaderm

12) You have a #3 knife handle on your back table. Which of these blade sizes would *not* fit on it?
   a. 10
   b. 11
   c. 15
   d. 20

13) Ioban <u>cannot</u> be used on a patient with a(n) _____ allergy.
   a. iodine
   b. latex
   c. wheat
   d. sulfa

14) DuraPrep contains both iodophor (Betadine) and _____.
   a. chlorhexidine
   b. detergent
   c. alcohol
   d. soap

15) Specimens for frozen section should be sent to the laboratory in:
   a. a suction trap
   b. a specimen container with formalin
   c. a dry specimen container
   d. a culture tube

16) Another name for a Glassman viscera retainer is a(n):
   a. isolation bag
   b. fish
   c. swab
   d. blade

17) Raney clips are used to hold _____ tissue.
   a. bowel
   b. bone
   c. scalp
   d. spine

18) The surgeon is performing a transurethral resection of the prostate using a resectoscope. Which of the following solutions will most likely be used for intraoperative irrigation?
   a. glycine
   b. sterile water
   c. sterile saline
   d. Iodophor

19) You are scrubbed on a vascular procedure and intraoperative angiography is anticipated. Which of the following will you most likely have on your sterile field?
   a. indigo carmen
   b. methylene blue
   c. Omnipaque
   d. gentian violet

20) Polymethyl methacrylate is also known as:
   a. bone wax
   b. heparin
   c. thrombin
   d. bone cement

21) Sterile mineral oil would most likely be used during which type of procedure?
   a. open reduction internal fixation of an ankle
   b. skin graft
   c. appendectomy
   d. cholecystectomy

CHAPTER 3

Tubes, Drains, Catheters and Postop Splints

DRAINS

Drains are placed in the surgical wound to remove blood, fluid, air or, in some cases, pus. This allows the wound to heal without formation of fluid pockets, air pockets or hematomas.

Drains can be *passive,* meaning that they create an opening from inside the wound to outside the body, or they can be *active,* meaning that they drain the wound using negative pressure (suction). Passive drains are simple and generally are used in situations in which minimal drainage is expected. They use gravity to drain the wound, either into an attached container or into the dressing. Active (or suction) drains are used for moderate or large amounts of drainage. They always require the use of a collection device to create the negative pressure. All drains are disposable, single patient use items.

This chapter covers passive drains followed by a section on active drains.

Passive Drains

Penrose

The Penrose drain is a soft tube of rubber or silicone placed into a wound to create a conduit for drainage to reach the body surface (see Fig. 3-1). It is not connected to a collection device; instead, it drains the fluid directly into the dressing.

Penrose drains also can be moistened with saline and used to retract delicate structures (e.g., the esophagus or spermatic cord) during surgery. They are available in 12-, 18- and 36-inch lengths but can easily be cut to the desired length. Available widths are ¼, ⅜, ½, ⅝, ¾, ⅞ and 1 inch.

A type of drain that is similar to the Penrose and used less often is the *cigarette drain.* This drain looks like a Penrose but has a gauze strip in the center of the tube.

Biliary T-Tube

As the name implies, the T-tube is a latex tube shaped like the letter T. It is placed in the biliary tract after surgery to facilitate drainage of bile from the common bile duct. This type of drain is often used during open gallbladder or common bile duct surgeries. The T-tube is attached to a collection device known as a *bile bag* (see Fig. 3-2). The bile is collected in the bile bag to allow for visualization and measurement. T-tubes come in sizes ranging from 5 Fr to 24 Fr. They usually have

an 11- to 12-inch stem with a 5- or 12-inch crossbar but can be cut to the desired size.

Tympanostomy Tube

A tympanostomy tube (also known as a *pressure equalization* or *PE tube*) is used to ventilate and equalize pressure in the middle ear as well as to allow drainage to escape. This type of drain is used to treat recurrent ear infections. It is inserted through a small incision in the tympanic membrane (ear drum) called a *myringotomy.* There are several styles of tubes; the most popular

FIGURE 3-1 Penrose drain.

FIGURE 3-2 T-tube and bile bag.

are the *grommet, button* and *bobbin* (see Fig. 3-3). These drains are extremely small (only millimeters) and must be handled carefully with micro alligator forceps.

Active Drains

Jackson-Pratt Drain

A Jackson-Pratt (JP) drain is a thin radiopaque tube with multiple drainage holes that is connected to clear plastic tubing (see Fig. 3-4). The drain part is placed inside the wound and the plastic tubing is on the outside of the body. The tubing is connected to a separate collection device known as a *bulb reservoir*. The drain is connected, the empty bulb squeezed to get the air out and the reservoir cap is closed. This creates gentle suction that pulls fluid and blood out of the wound.

A JP drain can be left in the wound for as little as 24 hours or up to several weeks. It is removed once the wound drainage subsides. The cap on the reservoir can be opened to allow for emptying the drainage.

JP drains can be used following many types of surgery including general, orthopedic, plastic, neurological, gynecological, cardiovascular and head/neck procedures. They are available in 7-mm, 10-mm and 15-mm diameters.

Blake Drains

A Blake drain is a radiopaque silicone drain that consists of four channels along the sides and a solid core center (see Fig. 3-4). The drain comes attached to silicone tubing. This drain works similar to a JP drain in that the Blake drain is placed in the wound and the tubing is outside the body. The Blake drain is attached to a *bulb reservoir* (see Fig. 3-4) in the same fashion as the JP drain.

Blake drains can be used following a variety of surgeries including orthopedic, cardiovascular, plastic, neurological, gynecological, head/neck and general procedures. The Blake drain is available in a flat or round shape. The flat Blake drain is available in 7 mm or 10 mm. The round style is available in 10 mm, 15 mm, 19 mm or 24 mm.

Hemovac

The Hemovac drain (also known as a *spring action drain*) consists of a round collection reservoir with three springs inside it that attaches to a multi-holed silicone drain (see Fig. 3-5). The drain is attached to the collection reservoir, both sides of the reservoir are squeezed down nearly flat and the reservoir cap closed to create the vacuum (negative pressure). Hemovac collection devices have a capacity of 400 cc.

TLS Evacuated Tube Drain

The TLS evacuated tube drain (test tube type) consists of a silicone drain that is attached to clear glass vacuum test tubes (see Fig. 3-6). The drain kit comes with the drain and two 15-mL tubes. Extra tubes are available separately. These drains are designed specifically for use following surgery of the face or neck.

Drains are available in 7 mm or 10 mm with holes down the center or on the sides.

Chest Drainage Systems

Pleur-Evac

The Pleur-Evac is a widely used chest drainage system (see Fig. 3-7). This device consists of a three–chambered collection unit (originally modeled after the old three glass bottle system)

FIGURE 3-3 Tympanostomy tube.

FIGURE 3-4 JP and Blake drains and bulb reservoir.

FIGURE 3-5 Hemovac drain.

FIGURE 3-6 TLS evacuated tube drain.

that has two hoses: one attaches to the patient's chest tube and the other attaches to suction.

If the device is facing you, the chamber on the right is the chest drainage collection unit. The hose on the top of this chamber attaches to the patient's chest tube to allow blood and/or fluid to drain directly into the chamber. This chamber is marked with calibrations in milliliters (mL) to allow for measurement of drainage. The outside surface of this chamber can be written on to allow marking of date and time drainage is checked so that the amount of drainage the patient is putting out can be measured.

The middle chamber is the water seal chamber. This chamber allows air to exit the pleural space with exhalation and prevents air from entering the pleural space with inhalation. This chamber must be filled with sterile fluid up to the 2-cm water level marking. To maintain this water seal, the Pleur-Evac needs always to be kept in an upright position and the water level monitored (fluid can evaporate and may need to be refilled). If there is no air leak, the water level in this chamber should rise with inspiration and fall with expiration, reflecting normal pressure changes in the pleural cavity. Exceptionally high negative pressure readings can be caused by respiratory distress, crying, decreased or disconnected suction or stripping the chest tube. High pressures are indicated by a rising water level in the small arm of the chamber.

The left hand chamber is the suction control chamber. In older models, the chamber is "wet," requiring it to be filled to a specified line with sterile fluid. In newer models, the suction control chamber is "dry," thus not requiring fluid to be added. The dry models have several advantages over the older "wet" models:

1. There is no fluid bubbling; therefore, they are much quieter (a plus for patient and roommate for whom the continuous bubbling could be irritating).
2. There is no fluid that can evaporate, causing decreased suction levels.
3. Higher suction levels can be achieved.
4. They are easier to set up.

The hose on the top of this chamber is connected to the suction. Pleur-Evacs come with a preset level of −20 cm of water for suction but can be set to −10 cm, −15 cm, −30 cm and −40 cm (refer to manufacturer's instructions). Conditions in which the suction may need to be adjusted higher (−30 cm or −40 cm) include empyema, a large air leak from the lung surface or anticipated problems with lung re-expansion.

Chest tube drainage systems are used for treatment of pneumothorax (spontaneous or traumatic) or for re-expansion of the lung(s) and re-establishment of proper pleural cavity pressures following cardiothoracic surgery. Chest tubes are placed at the end of the surgery and the Pleur-Evac is attached.

Chest Tubes

Chest tubes are flexible, clear plastic drains that are inserted into the chest cavity. They are used to drain air, fluid, blood or pus into a water seal collection device, such as a Pleur-Evac. Depending on the circumstances, more than one chest tube may be required on the same side, or they may be required bilaterally. Chest tubes have holes (known as *eyes*) in the end that is inserted into the chest to allow for flow of drainage into the tube, and the other end is attached to the collection device hose adapter (see Fig. 3-8). Chest tubes come with a sharp metal trocar that can be used to insert the chest tube. Whether

FIGURE 3-7 A) Dry Pleur-Evac. B) Wet Pleur-Evac.

or not the trocar is used depends on the circumstances and surgeon preference.

Chest tubes are generally secured in place with a purse-string suturing method to enable easier wound closure upon removal of the tube.

Caution: Chest tubes should NOT be "stripped" to maintain patency. Stripping of chest tubes can cause pressures of −400 cm or higher!

Chest tubes are available in a variety of diameters. The size used depends on patient size and circumstances. Generally, a smaller tube (18 to 22 Fr) is used to treat an adult with a pneumothorax, whereas a larger tube (26 to 32 Fr) is used in the presence of a hemothorax (blood) or empyema (pus).

Heimlich Chest Drain Valve

Manufactured by BD Bard-Parker, the Heimlich chest drain valve (see Fig. 3-9) is a device that can be used in place of a traditional water seal drainage system such as Pleur-Evac in some circumstances. The Heimlich system consists of rubber flutter leaflets encased in a plastic chamber with adapters on both ends. The proximal adapter is attached to the patient's chest tube while the distal one is attached to tubing leading to a plastic drainage bag or regulated suction, if desired. The device is easily portable and can function in any position.

According to the manufacturer, uses of the Heimlich device include treatment of spontaneous pneumothorax, recurrent pleural effusion, open thoracotomy and traumatic hemopneumothorax. (See www.bd.com for additional information.)

Ventricular (Cerebrospinal Fluid) Drains

External Ventricular Drain

An external ventricular drain (EVD) is used to drain excess cerebrospinal fluid (CSF) from the brain ventricles into a bag outside the body (see Fig. 3-10). These drains are external, as compared with ventricular shunts that shunt the CSF internally into the peritoneum or heart atrium.

FIGURE 3-9 Heimlich chest valve.

External drains collect the excess CSF and they can be used to take pressure measurements in the brain to check for increased intracranial pressure, a potentially life-threatening problem. The collection devices with these systems are calibrated in milliliters and are clear to allow for visualization and measurement of the CSF.

Conditions that could cause increased intracranial pressure and therefore necessitate the use of an EVD are obstructive tumors, serious head injury or a burst aneurysm.

Ventricular Shunt

A ventricular shunt (see Fig. 3-10) is an internal drain that shunts the excess CSF from the ventricles to either the peritoneum (ventriculoperitoneal shunt) or the heart atrium (ventriculoatrial shunt). These devices are used to treat hydrocephalus.

Hydrocephalus is a condition that results in an increased amount of CSF in the ventricles. This condition can be congenital (present at birth) or acquired. Congenital hydrocephalus can be caused by infection (e.g., rubella), congenital malformations or hemorrhaging in the brain. Acquired hydrocephalus can happen at any age and may be caused by hemorrhage, trauma, tumor, cysts or infection (e.g., bacterial meningitis or abscess formation).

FIGURE 3-8 Chest tube with trocar.

FIGURE 3-10 External ventricular drain and ventricular shunts.

There are many types of shunts; you need to be familiar with the types that your institution uses. As with any implant, these shunts should be handled as little as possible and kept away from lint and dust. Absolute adherence to aseptic technique is essential. One of the major complications of this type of shunt is infection, which can lead to patient death.

Autotransfusion

Autotransfusion is the reinfusion of the patient's own blood or blood products. The patient may donate blood or blood products before having surgery, or blood may be collected intraoperatively or postoperatively and then reinfused. The intraoperative and postoperative blood collection and reinfusion devices are covered in this section.

Why Reinfuse?

Reinfusing the patient's own blood is preferable to a donor transfusion because it eliminates the danger of blood incompatibility and possible disease transmission. In some cases, patients who refuse a blood transfusion from an outside source may be willing to accept an autotransfusion.

There are times when you are not able to collect the patient's blood and reinfuse it. The patient's blood should not be reinfused if:

- The patient has a known infection (localized or systemic).
- The blood has been exposed to antibiotics (including antibiotic irrigating solutions) or collagen hemostatic agents; these can cause blood to coagulate in the machine.
- The blood has mixed with amniotic fluid or gastric or bowel contents.

There are several types of devices that can be used to collect the blood, process it and ready it for reinfusion back into the patient. The following sections describe the most common types of machines and their uses.

Cell Saver or Cell Salvager

The cell saver or cell salvager allows the blood to be suctioned directly from the surgical field into the machine (see Fig. 3-11). In addition to suctioning blood directly from the field, bloody sponges can be soaked in a basin of saline and the bloody saline suctioned into the machine. The machine filters and anticoagulates the blood and fluid, readying it for intravenous reinfusion back to the patient. This process causes little or no harm to the red blood cells.

The cell saver is able to process large quantities of blood and irrigation fluid and is used when a large blood loss is possible, such as in cases of ruptured spleen or large blood vessel, major spinal surgery, major orthopedic procedures or multiple traumas with suspected major bleeding.

One major disadvantage to the cell saver device is that it may require a dedicated operator to run it. Check your institution's policy about who can operate a cell saver.

FIGURE 3-11 Cell saver machine.

OrthoPat Blood Salvaging Device

This blood salvaging device is designed to be used during orthopedic procedures in which blood loss may be sufficient enough to require transfusion (e.g., total hip replacement).

The OrthoPat can be used postoperatively to collect and prepare blood for reinfusion. Instead of suctioning blood from the surgical field, the OrthoPat device is attached to the drain (see Fig. 3-12). The blood is drained from the surgical field into the machine, where it is cleansed and prepared for reinfusion.

This device is capable of processing smaller amounts of blood and fluid than a cell saver and is designed for use during orthopedic procedures in which blood loss is intermittent. It is *not* designed to be used for major blood loss such as occurs with a ruptured spleen or bleeding aorta. One major advantage is that the machine is fully automated and can be monitored by the circulating personnel; it does not require a dedicated operator. Refer to the manufacturer's instructions for set-up, use and troubleshooting.

Autotransfusion Drains

The simplest of autotransfusion devices are the postoperative collection drains. These devices are closed collection systems that use a three-spring evacuator (similar to a Hemovac drain) or controlled wall suction to suction blood from the surgical wound postoperatively and collect it for possible reinfusion back to the patient. These devices contain filters within the collection chamber to filter out clots and debris. They have access ports to allow for the addition of anticoagulant medication.

FIGURE 3–12 OrthoPat device.

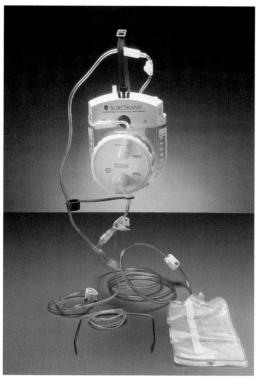

FIGURE 3–13 Suretrans system.

The advantages to these drains are that they are easy to set up and use; they are closed systems, thus decreasing the chance of staff exposure to blood; and they are relatively inexpensive when compared with other reinfusion technology. The transfer of the fluid into the reinfusion bag is easily accomplished (usually the push of a button or lever) and you only need one device per patient (they can be used to collect and reinfuse multiple times). The disadvantages are that they can be used postoperatively only (not intraoperatively) and they have a smaller collection capacity than some other devices.

As with any medical device, no matter which autotransfusion technology is being used you must make sure you are familiar with the device and how to use it *before* using it on your patient. If you are unfamiliar with the device, check your institution's procedure for its use and the manufacturer's instructions.

Suretrans

Manufactured by Davol, the Suretrans is an autotransfusion drain system (see Fig. 3-13) that allows blood to be collected and re-infused back to the patient after orthopedic surgery. Suction is created with a spring action evacuator (similar to a Hemovac) that is attached to the collection reservoir. The 800-mL collection reservoir is clear (to allow for visualization and measuring of drainage) and contains a filter and blood transfer button. If re-infusion of the blood is desired, the blood transfer button allows the blood to go from the reservoir to the 1000-mL blood bag. The blood can then be reinfused according to institutional policy. The reinfusion takes place from the blood bag, allowing

the evacuator to continue working to collect drainage while reinfusion is going on.

ConstaVac CBCII system

Manufactured by Stryker the ConstaVac CBC system is an autotransfusion drain system that allows blood to be collected and reinfused back to the patient after orthopedic surgery. The system consists of a clear 800-mL reservoir that contains a filter for blood collection and a reinfusion bag (see Fig. 3-14). The drain is attached to the reservoir, which has a variable vacuum setting. To transfer the blood from the reservoir to the blood bag, depress the lever. The blood in the blood bag can then be reinfused according to institutional policy. The reinfusion takes place from the blood bag, allowing the evacuator to continue working to collect drainage while reinfusion is going on.

GASTROINTESTINAL TUBES

Nasogastric Tubes

Nasogastric tubes are inserted through the nose into the back of the throat, down the esophagus and into the stomach. These tubes are used most commonly to decompress the stomach but can be used for gastric lavage (in drug overdoses), for enteral feedings, or to obtain specimens for analysis. These tubes are for short-term use (usually less than 6 weeks). Prolonged usage could lead to necrosis of the nasal septum.

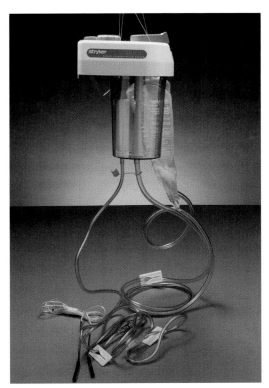

FIGURE 3-14 ConstaVac CBC system.

The *Levin tube* is another type of nasogastric tube. The Levin tube is a single-lumen tube made of rubber or PVC plastic (see Fig. 3-16). The plastic tube is used more commonly because it contains a radiopaque strip to allow for radiographic confirmation of tube placement. It is used to aspirate stomach contents or instill medication. This type of tube is attached to intermittent low suction. Levin tubes are 50 inches long and are available in 6-Fr to 24-Fr diameters.

Gastrostomy Tubes

A gastrostomy tube is placed, endoscopically or surgically, directly into the patient's stomach. These tubes can be temporary or permanent. They are used for patients who cannot swallow correctly or continually aspirate food, for people who cannot take in enough food by mouth to keep well nourished and for infants with birth defects of the mouth or esophagus. The tube can be used to instill tube feedings and medication or to aspirate air and stomach contents.

Gastrostomy tubes come in a variety of styles but have some common features (see Fig. 3-17). All of them have a balloon at the distal tip that is inflated to keep them in place. They all have at least one port to allow instillation of enteral feedings, fluids or medications. Some tubes have two or more

The *Salem sump tube* is the most widely used nasogastric tube. It is made of polyvinyl chloride (PVC) plastic. This tube is double-lumened to allow for suction drainage and air ventilation. The drainage lumen is usually connected to continuous low suction. The ventilation lumen helps to keep the tube away from the stomach wall and to decrease the chance of damage to the mucosa. If irrigation is necessary, the ventilation port can be used for this purpose. A radiopaque line runs the length of the tube to allow for radiographic conformation of placement. Salem sump tubes are available in 24-inch length (for pediatric patients), 36- and 48-inch lengths (see Fig. 3-15). The available diameters range from 6 Fr to 18 Fr.

FIGURE 3-16 Levin tube.

FIGURE 3-15 Salem sump tubes.

FIGURE 3-17 Regular gastrostomy.

ports so that feedings do not have to be interrupted to give medications or to allow for gastric decompression. Gastrostomy tubes are made of silicone and have a radiopaque strip to allow for radiographic confirmation of placement. The feeding port is flexible to accommodate a variety of catheter tip syringes. The most common sizes of these tubes are 12-Fr (pediatric) through 24-Fr diameters.

One common style of gastrostomy tube is known as a *feeding peg* or *button*. This style of tube is made to fit closely to the skin surface, making it less noticeable under clothing. These are generally used if long-term or permanent use is anticipated. These tubes are available in 14-Fr through 24-Fr diameters, in a variety of stoma lengths (1.5 to 4.0 cm) to accommodate most patients.

Nasointestinal Tubes

Nasointestinal tubes are longer than nasogastric tubes and are designed to treat a small bowel obstruction (see Fig. 3-18). They have a weighted distal end and rely on peristalsis to move them along the intestinal tract to relieve the obstruction.

The older styles, such as the single-lumen *Cantor* or *Harris* tube or double-lumen *Miller-Abbott* tube have a mercury-filled balloon at the distal end. These tubes are not commonly used because there is a chance that the balloon might rupture, and mercury would spill into the patient's body.

The newer style nasointestinal tubes have a tungsten-weighted distal end rather than the mercury-filled balloon, making them safer to use. Newer styles include the newer *Miller-Abbott* and *Andersen* tubes. Nasointestinal tubes are available in 10-Fr (pediatric) through 22-Fr diameters.

Sengstaken-Blakemore Tube

The Sengstaken-Blakemore is a triple-lumen tube used to tamponade bleeding from esophageal varices. Two of the lumens are used to inflate balloons that provide pressure to the bleeding varices, and the third lumen is used to drain gastric contents.

This tube is placed as an emergency measure when bleeding is too heavy to be stopped by the use of medication. It is a temporary measure; prolonged use has been associated with ulceration or rupture of the esophagus and stomach. Placement of the tube can be difficult, and airway obstruction could result if it is inadvertently placed in the trachea.

URETHRAL CATHETERS

Urethral catheters come in two major categories: indwelling (*retention*) and straight (*nonretention*). Generally, urethral catheters are used to drain urine from the bladder, but indwelling catheters can be placed in a cavity as a drain and nonretaining catheters can be used as irrigation devices in ducts or body cavities.

The diameter of urethral catheters is measured in French (Fr) sizes. The larger the number, the larger the diameter of the catheter (e.g., 8 Fr is a very narrow catheter generally used for small children; 32 Fr is a large diameter catheter). The most common sizes of catheters are 14 Fr, 16 Fr and 18 Fr.

In the past, all urethral catheters were made of rubber. In light of the growing concern over latex exposure and the increasing number of people who are latex allergic, most styles of catheters are available now made with nonlatex material (usually silicone).

This section covers the types and uses of the most common indwelling and straight urethral catheters.

Indwelling (Retention) Catheters

Foley Catheters

When we think of an indwelling urethral catheter, the Foley catheter is the one that comes to mind. It is the most common one used. A Foley catheter has a balloon at one end that can be inflated to hold the catheter in place. The balloon has either a 5-cc or a 30-cc capacity (see Fig. 3-19). The 5-cc balloon is used simply to hold the catheter in place. A Foley with a 30-cc balloon is used to maintain hemostasis (e.g., after transurethral resection of the prostate [TURP]).

Foley catheters can have a two-way or a three-way system. The two-way system is the common Foley catheter that we all think of; it has one port through which to inflate the balloon

FIGURE 3–18 Nasointestinal tube.

General Catheterization Guidelines

There are several important things to remember before inserting any urethral catheter:

- Before opening the catheter or catheter kit, check patient allergies. If the patient has a latex sensitivity or allergy, make sure you have a nonlatex catheter.

- Urethral catheterization is a STERILE procedure. Be sure to maintain strict aseptic technique when handling and inserting a catheter. Failure to maintain asepsis could result in a urinary tract infection for the patient and possible increased hospital stay or other complications.

- Catheters are one time use. If you contaminate the catheter while trying to insert it or if the catheter selected is the wrong size, you need to get a new one.

- Foley catheter balloons should be inflated and deflated *prior to* use to check for leaks, holes, failure to deflate and other problems.

FIGURE 3-19 Foley catheters with 5-cc and 30-cc balloons inflated.

Malecot catheters

The Malecot catheter is another type of self-retaining urethral catheter. Instead of using a balloon, the tip of the Malecot has either two or four wings that expand out to hold it in place (see Fig. 3-21). The most common Malecot catheter sizes are 12 Fr through 18 Fr. In addition to being used to drain urine from the bladder, Malecot catheters can be inserted into the stomach, to be used as a feeding tube, or into a wound or body cavity, to be used as a drain.

Pezzer Catheter

The Pezzer catheter, also known as a *mushroom catheter,* has a tip that resembles a mushroom cap that holds it in place (see Fig. 3-22). The mushroom-shaped tip has two holes to allow for drainage. Pezzer catheters are available in sizes 14 Fr through 32 Fr. Like other self-retaining catheters, the Pezzer can be used for bladder drainage, as a feeding tube or as a wound drain.

and one to which to hook a drainage bag (see Fig. 3-20). The three-way catheter has two drainage hookups—one for instilling irrigation fluids and one for a drainage bag—as well as a port to allow for balloon inflation (see Fig. 3-20). The three-way Foley is used when continuous or intermittent bladder irrigation is desired.

Foley catheters have several uses:

- Long-term drainage of the bladder
- Decompression of the bladder during surgery to decrease the chance of bladder injury
- Continuous bladder irrigation
- Blood clot evacuation
- Measurement and tracking of urinary output
- Possible drainage of a body cavity (e.g., can be used as a chest tube)

FIGURE 3-21 Four-wing Malecot self-retaining catheter.

FIGURE 3-20 Two-way Foley and three-way Foley catheters.

FIGURE 3-22 Pezzer catheter.

Urinary Drainage Bags

All self-retaining catheters need to be attached to a drainage bag. There are two types of bags: a leg bag that is often used during the day when the person is up and about and a larger bag that is used when the patient is in the hospital or in bed at night (sometimes referred to as a *nighttime bag*).

The leg bag is a small bag that attaches around the upper leg with two straps: one at the top of the bag and one at the bottom (see Fig. 3-23A). The leg bag is worn under clothing to conceal it from view when the person is out in public or participating in activities. It allows the person greater freedom because he or she does not have to carry a bag around. Leg bags have a smaller capacity (anywhere from 450 cc to 1300 cc; most common are 600 cc to 800 cc) and need to be emptied more frequently than the larger nighttime bags. Most leg bags have a hard plastic valve at the bottom for ease of emptying.

The larger bag (or nighttime bag) is the bag most frequently used in the operating room. The self-retaining catheter is attached to the bag to allow the bladder to continuously drain. Urinary output and color can be monitored during the procedure and postoperatively. This type of bag is less convenient if the patient is going to be going home with an indwelling catheter as it cannot be concealed under clothing and must be carried around by hand. Patients who go home with an indwelling catheter and leg bag also will have this larger drainage bag to use at night (so that they do not have to wake up in the night to empty it).

Larger urinary drainage bags are available in 2000-cc to 4000-cc capacity, with or without a urometer attached (see Fig. 3-23B). A urometer is a 350-cc to 500-cc device that allows for more careful monitoring of urinary output over shorter time intervals (e.g., anesthesia may want to use this type of bag for someone undergoing major surgery for whom they need to monitor hourly urine outputs). The urine flows into the urometer and the measurement is taken and then the urometer is emptied into the larger bag.

Nonretaining (Straight) Catheters

Nonretaining catheters, also known as *straight catheters,* are used temporarily to drain the bladder or to irrigate a duct. These catheters do not have balloons or wings to hold them in place. Drainage bags are unnecessary because the catheter does not stay in. The straight catheter is inserted, the bladder is drained and the catheter is immediately removed. They may be inserted at the beginning of the surgical procedure to drain the bladder when an empty bladder is desirable but ongoing bladder decompression is unnecessary.

Like indwelling catheters, straight catheters are sized according to the French gauge system. The most common sizes are 14 Fr and 16 Fr for adults, 10 Fr for children and 8 Fr for toddlers and some infants.

Coudé Catheter

A Coudé catheter is available in both self-retaining and nonretaining styles. This type of catheter has a curved, stiff tip that makes it easier to insert in the presence of an enlarged prostate or urethral stricture (see Fig. 3-24). This type of catheter is often used when attempts to insert a Foley catheter are unsuccessful.

Robinson Catheter

The Robinson catheter (also known as a *red rubber* or *straight cath*) is the most common nonretaining catheter. The tip is

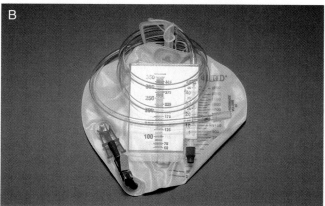

FIGURE 3-23 A) Urinary leg bag. B) Urinary drainage bag with a urometer attached.

FIGURE 3-24 Coudé catheter.

soft and rounded, with two opposing eyes for drainage (see Fig. 3-25). Robinson catheters are made of latex, thus the patient's allergies need to be checked prior to insertion. The most common sizes are 12 Fr through 18 Fr.

Ureteral Catheters

Ureteral catheters are narrow tubes inserted into the ureters with the use of a cystoscope. These catheters can be used to bypass a tumor or kidney stone, provide drainage of the ureter, keep the ureter open, instill contrast media, allow stones to pass, block the ureters during radiologic procedures or obtain specimens. Ureteral catheters may be inserted before open abdominal surgery to identify the ureter, thus decreasing the chance of injury to it.

Ureteral catheters are very narrow, generally ranging from 3-Fr to 6-Fr diameter (see Fig. 3-26). They are marked in centimeters to allow the surgeon to gauge how far they have been inserted. These catheters come in a variety of tip shapes: whistle, cone, open end, spiral, round, angled and wedge (looks like a Pezzer tip). The type of catheter the surgeon selects depends on the purpose for which it is being used. For example, a wedge tip may be used during a retrograde pyelogram, whereas an open-end tip is used for drainage or navigating a tortuous ureter.

Ureteral Stents

Some patients have the ureteral catheter left in place postoperatively to allow for healing. This is known as a *stent* and it can be attached to a urinary drainage bag. Two of the most common types are the J stent and the pigtail (see Figs. 3-27 and 3-28). Both catheters have a spiral shape to the end, which helps to hold them in place in the ureter. The length of time a stent is left in place depends on how long the healing process takes; it can be anywhere from days to months (or even years). If the stent is to be left in long-term, the patient may need to come back into surgery periodically to have it changed.

Many stents come with a tether attached. A tether is a long strand of material attached to the stent that aids in the manipulation or removal of the stent. The surgeon may choose to leave the tether attached (in which case it is often secured to the inside of the upper thigh) or cut it off.

FIGURE 3-25 Robinson catheter.

FIGURE 3-27 J stent.

FIGURE 3-26 Different types of ureteral catheters.

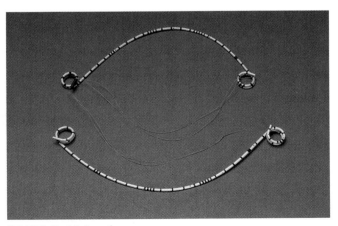

FIGURE 3-28 Pigtail stent.

SPLINTS

Name: Philadelphia collar

Alias: rigid cervical brace

Use: supports neck post cervical injury or surgery

Features: rigid foam construction; two pieces: front and back

Additional Information: available with hole in the front for tracheostomies or with solid front; available in extra small through large sizes; collar height varies from 2.25 inches (extra small) through 5.25 inches (large)

Philadelphia collar
Soft collar

Name: soft cervical collar

Alias: none

Use: supports minor cervical injuries or acts as a transition collar between a more rigid collar and no collar

Features: soft 1-inch thick foam; easily contours to neck

Additional Information: available in small, medium, large and extra large sizes; collar height varies from 3 inches (small) to 4.25 inches (extra large)

Name: knee immobilizer

Alias: knee splint

Use: immobilizes knee in a straight position post injury or surgery

Features: Velcro straps for easy adjustment; padded inside; cut out area fits over knee

Additional Information: available in 12- through 26-inch lengths; available in sizes extra small through universal

Name: hip abduction pillow

Alias: none

Use: provides hip abduction following hip surgery

Features: foam pillow; foam straps help to keep it positioned correctly

Additional Information: available in small (12.5-inch base × 18-inch length) or large (17-inch base × 24-inch length)

Name: abdominal binder

Alias: none

Use: provides postoperative abdominal support

Features: stretchable to accommodate a variety of abdominal girths; Velcro closure

Additional Information: available in small, medium, large and universal sizes

Name: sling

Alias: none

Use: provides support to arm and limits mobility post trauma or surgery

Features: adjustable shoulder strap; padded arm rest to support arm

Additional Information: many styles of sling are available; many slings have a swathe without the waist strap; most types available in adult and pediatric sizes

Name: sling and swathe

Alias: shoulder immobilizer

Use: immobilizes shoulder post trauma or surgery

Features: arm is placed in sling and strap goes around waist to hold the arm close to the body; adjustable waist and shoulder straps

Additional Information: many styles of sling and swathe are available; most are available in sizes small through extra large; some have padded waist and shoulder straps

Name: Post-surgical bra

Alias: breast support

Use: holds dressings in place; provides compression and support following breast surgery

Features: front closure; expandable fabric to allow for swelling

Additional Information: available in sizes extra small to XX-large

Q&A Surgical Session Review

1) A _____ drain does not have an attached fluid collection device.
   a. Pleur-Evac
   b. Hemovac
   c. Penrose
   d. TLS

2) A Heimlich valve is used to drain air from the:
   a. abdomen
   b. chest
   c. knee joint
   d. pelvic cavity

3) A Levin is a type of:
   a. nasogastric tube
   b. chest tube
   c. wound drain
   d. tracheostomy tube

4) A Malecot is a type of:
   a. nasogastric tube
   b. wound drain
   c. ventricular drain
   d. urinary catheter

5) The urologist is having trouble catheterizing an elderly male patient due to an enlarged prostate. Which type of catheter is he most likely to ask you to have available?
   a. Robinson
   b. three-way Foley
   c. Coudé
   d. Salem

6) Your patient has had anterior cervical surgery. Which of the following splints might the surgeon apply at the end of the case?
   a. sling
   b. sling with swathe
   c. abductor pillow
   d. Philadelphia collar

7) A Suretrans drain is most likely to be used following what type of surgery?
   a. craniotomy
   b. total knee
   c. radical neck
   d. total abdominal hysterectomy

8) Filiformes and followers are used for what type of procedure?
   a. urethral stricture dilation
   b. wound irrigation and drainage
   c. intubation
   d. gastric decompression

9) A TLS drain could be used following surgery on all of these areas *except:*
   a. foot
   b. face
   c. breast
   d. knee

10) A JP drain is another name for a:
    a. Jackman-Pratt
    b. Jackson-Pratt
    c. Jackson-Prett
    d. Jackman-Prett

11) A Salem sump is a common type of:
    a. urinary catheter
    b. tracheostomy tube
    c. nasogastric tube
    d. endotracheal tube

12) Your patient has undergone an open rotator cuff repair. Which splint might be used to immobilize the shoulder postoperatively?
    a. regular sling
    b. sling and swathe
    c. soft collar
    d. Philadelphia collar

13) J and "double pigtail" are types of:
    a. wound drains
    b. Foley catheters
    c. ureteral stents
    d. chest tubes

CHAPTER 4

Sutures and Suture Needles

COMPARISON OF SUTURE MATERIALS

Sutures are composed of various materials, which make them suitable for certain procedures or tissues. Tables 4–1, 4–2 and 4–3 allow you to compare suture materials used by various manufacturers. Approximate wound support times are listed with the absorbable sutures to allow for further comparisons.

COMPONENTS OF SUTURE PACKAGING

You can judge some things by their covers. Shown here are the components that make up the information found on the outer packaging of the suture material produced by four major suture manufacturers.

Ethicon (see Fig. 4-1)
Manufacturer's Major Suture Brands
- Ethilon
- Surgical Stainless Steel
- Nurolon
- Mersilene
- Prolene
- Ethibond
- Silk (Mersilk)
- Surgical Gut (Plain)
- Surgical Gut (Chromic)
- Vicryl
- Vicryl Plus
- Vicryl Rapide
- Monocryl
- Panacryl

Syneture (see Fig. 4-2)
Manufacturer's Major Suture Brands
- Dermalon
- TiCron
- Novafil
- SurgiDac
- Vascufil
- Novafil
- Surgipro
- Flexon

Table 4-1 Non-absorbable Sutures

SUTURE MATERIAL	SYNETURE PRODUCT (US SUTURE/DAVIS AND GECK)	ETHICON PRODUCT
Monofilament nylon	Dermalon; Monosof	Ethilon
Braided nylon	Surgilon	Nurolon
Braided polyester (uncoated)	Surgidac	Mersilene
Braided polyester (coated)	Ti Cron	Ethibond Excel
Monofilament polybutester	Novafil	—
Monofilament polybutester (coated)	Vascufil	—
Monofilament polypropylene	Surgipro; Surgipro II	Prolene
Hexafluoropropylene VDF	—	Pronova Poly
Monofilament steel	Steel	Surgical Stainless Steel
Multistrand steel	Flexon	Surgical Stainless Steel
Silk	Sofsilk	Silk; Perma-Hand

Table 4-2 Other NonAbsorbable Sutures

SUTURE MATERIAL	SUTURE NAME AND MANUFACTURER
Monofilament nylon (ophthalmic)	Alcon Nylon Suture (made by Alcon)
Twisted silk (ophthalmic)	Silk suture (made by Alcon)
Monofilament polypropylene (ophthalmic)	Polypropylene suture (made by Alcon)
Braided polyester (ophthalmic)	Polyester suture (made by Alcon)
Monofilament suture coated with polycaprolate	BioSorb and BioSorb C (made by Alcon); BioSorb C also available as a braided suture
Monofilament PTFE (polytetrafluoroethylene)	Gore-Tex (made by Gore Medical)

- Sofsilk
- Plain Gut
- Chromic Gut
- Maxon
- Dexon
- Biosyn
- Polysorb
- Caprosyn

FIGURE 4-1 Ethicon suture package components.

Gore Medical (see Fig. 4-3)

Manufacturer's Major Suture Brands
- Gore-Tex cardiovascular suture

Alcon (see Fig. 4-4)

Manufacturer's Major Suture Brands
- Alcon Nylon, Polyester, Polypropylene and Silk ophthalmic sutures
- BioSorb
- BioSorb C

Table 4-3 Absorbable Sutures

SUTURE MATERIAL	SYNETURE PRODUCT (US SUTURE/ DAVIS AND GECK)	ETHICON PRODUCT
Gut fiber	Plain Gut (7–10 day wound support)	Surgical Gut– Plain (7–10 day wound support)
Gut fiber with chromium salt	Chromic Gut; Mild Chromic Gut (10–14 day wound support)	Surgical Gut Chromic (10–14 day wound support)
Synthetic monofilament polyglyconate	Maxon, Maxon Plus (6–week wound support)	—
Monofilament synthetic polyester (polyglytone 6211)	Caprosyn (10–day wound support)	—
Coated glycolic acid polymer	Dexon II, Dexon S (3–week wound support)	—
Monofilament polyester	Biosyn (3–week wound support)	—
Monofilament polydioxanone	—	PDS (up to 6–weeks' wound support)
Monofilament poliglecaprone	—	Monocryl (7–14 day wound support)
Braided copolymer of lactide and glycolide	Polysorb (3–week wound support)	Panacryl (up to 6 month wound support)
Braided polyglactin 910	—	Vicryl Rapide (7–10 day wound support)
		Vicryl (2–3 week wound support)

Sources: *Ethicon Wound Closure Manual* (2004); www.syneture.com; www.Alcon.com.

FIGURE 4-2 Syneture suture package components.

FIGURE 4-4 Alcon suture package components.

FIGURE 4-3 Gore Medical suture package components.

SUTURE SIZING

Sutures come in a variety of sizes (known as the *gauge*). Suture gauges range from 5 (heaviest suture) down to 11-0 (thinner than a strand of hair).

5 4 3 2 1 0 2-0 3-0 4-0 5-0 6-0 7-0 8-0 9-0 10-0 11-0

Heavy   Very Fine
Suture   Suture

The gauge of suture that a surgeon chooses depends on the thickness and type of tissue being sutured. The heavier sutures are used to approximate bone or are used to put retention sutures in an abdominal midline incision. Sutures that are 0 or 1 gauge are generally used on thick tissue (e.g., on abdominal muscle or fascia, during orthopedic surgery). Sutures in the 4-0 to 7-0 range generally are used in some plastic surgeries or in cardiovascular and vascular surgery. Sutures in the 8-0 to 11-0 range generally are used for surgery of the eye or in microsurgery procedures (e.g., microvascular, vasovasostomy) (see Fig. 4-5).

Suture Terms

When looking at suture, the following key terms that are important:

- *Absorbable:* This suture is capable of being absorbed by tissue in a given time frame, allowing the tissue time to heal itself. The time frame varies with each type of absorbable suture.
- *Non-absorbable:* This suture resists being absorbed by tissue. Used when a permanent suture is required or when the suture will be removed later (e.g., on the outside of the body).
- *Monofilament:* This suture consists of a single strand. This type of suture does not easily harbor bacteria and glides through tissue smoothly. The drawback to monofilament suture is that it can be harder to handle and does not hold a knot as well as a multifilament suture.
- *Multifilament:* This suture consists of more than one strand. The strands are either braided or twisted together. The advantages of multifilament suture are that it is easier to handle, holds knots better and has greater flexibility and tensile strength than monofilament

FIGURE 4-5 Suture thickness comparison.

suture. The disadvantage is that it can harbor bacteria and therefore should not be used in the presence of infection.

- *Braided:* The strands are intertwined.
- *Twisted:* The strands are twisted in the same direction.

- *Coated:* This suture is coated to ease handling and help reduce tissue drag (friction).
- *Natural:* This suture is made from naturally occurring plants or tissue (e.g., cotton suture).
- *Synthetic:* This suture is made from manufactured materials (e.g., nylon suture).

SUTURE

Name: AccuCount
Alias: needle counter
Use: holds used suture needles, knife blades and other sharps
Features: numbered foam insert; sticky surface on opposite side for blades
Additional Information: putting only one suture needle in each numbered space enables count to be accomplished more efficiently

Name: skin stapler
Alias: none
Use: closes skin incisions
Features: comes in regular and wide widths
Additional Information: available in a variety of styles

Name: retention suture bolster
Alias: bolster; booties
Use: sheaths the retention suture to avoid cutting the patient's skin
Features: made of rubber; surgical tubing
Additional Information: 12 to a package

Name: corkscrew suture anchor
Alias: none
Use: makes arthroscopic shoulder repairs
Features: corkscrew shaped anchor, two nonabsorbable polyester sutures (one green and one white)
Additional Information: comes as a disposable self-contained unit

Name: Mitek anchor

Alias: none

Use: makes rotator cuff repairs

Features: absorbable anchor with Panacryl and Ethibond sutures attached

Additional Information: comes as a disposable self-contained unit

Name: Dermabond

Alias: none

Use: approximates wound edges

Features: sterile, liquid topical skin adhesive

Additional Information: cannot be used on patients who have formaldehyde sensitivity

Name: Ethibond

Alias: none

Use: sutures general soft tissue

Features: nonabsorbable; braided

Additional Information: available in sizes 7-0 through 5; large diameter may be used for retention sutures; also available as ties

Name: stainless steel suture set

Alias: none

Use: repairs hernia, used for orthopedic procedures

Features: nonabsorbable, stainless steel suture material

Additional Information: comes with two sutures, one on a Keith (straight needle) and one on a tapercut needle; set includes a polypropylene button that can be used as a suture bolster

Name: EndoButton tape

Alias: none

Use: repairs tendon

Features: nonabsorbable; polyester fiber; blunt point needle

Additional Information: 5-mm wide

Name: Maxon

Alias: none

Use: closes wounds

Features: absorbable; monofilament

Additional Information: available in a variety of sizes and with a variety of needles; suture has "memory" (springs back into curls when removed from the package); scrub person needs to hold each end and give it one gentle pull outward before handing it to the surgeon

Name: Vicryl suture

Alias: none

Use: allows general soft tissue approximation

Features: braided; absorbable; tensile strength gone in 5 weeks

Additional Information: one of the most commonly used sutures; available in undyed or dyed (violet); sizes range from 8-0 though 2

Name: Vicryl reel

Alias: Ligapak

Use: ligates blood vessels or structures

Features: braided; absorbable; number of holes in the bottom of the reel indicates size (2 holes = 2-0, 4 holes = 4-0, and so on)

Additional Information: available in 2-0, 3-0 and 4-0 sizes; reel must be accounted for in your surgical count

Name: Novafil

Alias: none

Use: allows general tissue approximation

Features: monofilament; nonabsorbable

Additional Information: available in a variety of sizes; blue

Name: Panacryl

Alias: none

Use: sutures heavy tissue, ligaments, cartilage

Features: braided; undyed; absorbable

Additional Information: usually comes four sutures to a package

Name: Ethilon
Alias: nylon suture; skin suture
Use: closes skin; eye surgery
Features: monofilament; nonabsorbable; nylon fiber
Additional Information: available in black, green or undyed; available in sizes 11-0 to 2

Name: silk suture
Alias: none
Use: anastomoses bowel; secures drains
Features: braided; nonabsorbable; black
Additional Information: comes in a variety of sizes (9-0 to 5); 2-0 silk is the size most commonly used size for securing drains

Name: silk ties
Alias: none
Use: ligates blood vessels or structures
Features: braided; nonabsorbable; black
Additional Information: available in a variety of sizes (4-0 to 0 are the most common); come in 18-, 30- and 60-inch lengths or on reels

Name: Monocryl
Alias: none
Use: allows approximation of soft issue; not used for cardiovascular, neurological or ophthalmic tissue
Features: absorbable; monofilament; undyed or violet; tensile strength gone in 28 days
Additional Information: available in a variety of sizes (6-0 to 2); available with a variety of needles; suture has "memory" (springs back into curls when removed from the package); scrub person needs to hold each end and give it one gentle pull outward prior to handing it to the surgeon

Name: Vicryl ties
Alias: none
Use: ligates blood vessels or tissue
Features: braided; absorbable; violet
Additional Information: available in 18-, 27- and 30-inch lengths; available in a variety of sizes

Name: Alcon ophthalmic suture

Alias: none

Use: allows ophthalmic suturing

Features: monofilament; nonabsorbable; black nylon

Additional Information: double armed to allow for suturing in a circle; need to use Castroviejo or other microsurgery needle holder to handle

Name: Prolene

Alias: none

Use: allows general tissue approximation and ligation; often used in vascular surgery

Features: monofilament; nonabsorbable; may be clear or blue

Additional Information: available in sizes 10-0 to 2; suture has "memory" (springs back into curls when removed from the package); scrub person needs to hold each end and give it one gentle pull outward prior to handing it to the surgeon; smaller sizes available as double armed to allow for suturing in a circle around blood vessels

Name: PDS or PDS II

Alias: none

Use: allows soft tissue approximation except for adult cardiovascular or neural tissue; not for use in microsurgery

Features: monofilament; absorbable; clear or violet; absorption is complete within 6 months

Additional Information: available in sizes 9-0 to 2; suture has "memory" (springs back into curls when removed from the package); scrub person needs to hold each end and give it one gentle pull outward prior to handing it to the surgeon

Name: Gore-Tex suture

Alias: none

Use: commonly used in vascular cardiovascular surgery

Features: monofilament; nonabsorbable

Additional Information: available in a number of sizes; often comes double armed to allow for suturing in a circle around blood vessels

Name: Vicryl Rapide

Alias: none

Use: closure of skin and mucous membranes in cases in which 7 to 10 days of wound support is needed

Features: braided; absorbable; tensile strength completely gone in 10 to 14 days; undyed

Additional Information: available in sizes 5-0 to 1

Name: plain gut

Alias: none

Use: allows general tissue approximation; not for use in cardiovascular or neurosurgical procedures

Features: absorbable; made from collagen, which comes from beef or sheep intestines; packaged in alcohol to prevent suture from drying out

Additional Information: available in sizes 7-0 to 3; suture has "memory" (springs back into curls when removed from the package); scrub person needs to hold each end and give it one gentle pull outward prior to handing it to the surgeon; also available as ties

Name: chromic gut

Alias: surgical gut

Use: approximates general tissue; not for use in cardiovascular or neurosurgical procedures

Features: absorbable; made from collagen, which comes from beef or sheep intestines; packaged in alcohol to prevent suture from drying out; treated with chromium salts to delay absorption; *do not* use in patients with chromium allergies

Additional Information: available in sizes 7-0 to 3; suture has "memory" (springs back into curls when removed from the package); scrub person needs to hold each end and give it one gentle pull outward prior to handing it to the surgeon

Name: Mersilene

Alias: none

Use: allows general tissue approximation

Features: braided; nonabsorbable; may be undyed or green

Additional Information: available in sizes 11-0 and 10-0 (for use in ophthalmic and microsurgery procedures) and 6-0 to 5; also available as ties

Name: Dexon

Alias: none

Use: allows general tissue approximation

Features: braided; absorbable

Name: Nurolon

Alias: none

Use: approximates general tissue

Features: braided; nonabsorbable; nylon fiber

Additional Information: available in sizes 6-0 to 1

Name: stainless steel suture

Alias: none

Use: does the following: sternal closure, hernia repair, abdominal wound closure, tendon and cartilage repair

Features: nonabsorbable; should not be used in patients with stainless steel, nickel or chromium allergies

Additional Information: available in sizes 10-0 to 7

Name: Chromic Gut ties

Alias: surgical gut ties

Use: allows general tissue ligation; *do not* use in cardiovascular or neurosurgical procedures

Features: absorbable; made from collagen, which comes from beef or sheep intestines; packaged in alcohol to prevent suture from drying out; treated with chromium salts to delay absorption; *do not* use in patients with chromium allergies

Additional Information: available in sizes 3-0 to 0; available in 18- and 54-inch lengths; tie has "memory" (springs back into curls when removed from the package); scrub person needs to hold each end and give it one gentle pull outward prior to handing it to the surgeon

Name: Tevdek

Alias: none

Use: makes pursestring sutures in the aorta of adults; used in orthopedic procedures; sutures heavy tissue

Features: nonabsorbable; braided; green

Additional Information: available in a variety of sizes

Name: Pledgets

Alias: none

Use: exert pressure over small holes to prevent bleeding and promote clotting; prevent suture from tearing the tissue; used in some vascular procedures

Features: nonabsorbable

Additional Information: available in several sizes (3 × 7 mm pictured); fold the pledget in half and put the suture through the top half of the fold

Name: Ti Cron

Alias: none

Use: sutures heavy tissue (mainly in orthopedic surgery)

Features: nonabsorbable; braided; coated polyester; blue

Additional Information: available in a variety of sizes (2 and 5 are most popular sizes)

Name: Supramid Extra II

Alias: none

Use: used in plastic surgery, orthopedics, endodontics

Features: nonabsorbable; nylon fiber (composed of several fine nylon fibers enclosed in an outer smooth nylon shell)

Additional Information: comes as a looped cable; available in sizes 4-0 to 8

Name: Endoloop (PDS II)

Alias: looped suture

Use: ligates during endoscopic procedures

Features: needleless; comes in a single unit pack; 18 inches long

Additional Information: available in 0 Vicryl, 0 PDS II, 0 Ethibond, 0 Monocryl

Name: Endoknot

Alias: none

Use: used during endoscopic surgery

Features: straight taper needle attached to one end, the other end is attached to a scored plastic tubing that acts as a handle; 42 inches long

Additional Information: available in 0 Vicryl, 0 PDS II, 0 Ethibond, 2-0 Chromic

Name: Surgilene

Alias: none

Use: allows general tissue approximation

Features: nonabsorbable; monofilament; blue

Additional Information: available in sizes 5-0 to 7

SUTURE NEEDLE POINTS

The point or tip (see Figs. 4-6 and 4-7) is the first part of the needle to enter the tissue. The three most common types of tips are cutting, taper and blunt. Cutting needles generally are used to close skin or secure drains, taper needles generally are used on tissue inside the body cavity and blunt needles usually are used to suture organs (e.g., the liver).

The body (see Figs. 4-6 and 4-7) makes up the majority of the needle. This is the part that is held in the needle holder. Depending on the surgery, type of tissue and surgeon preference, the needle holder generally is placed on the distal half to one third of the body.

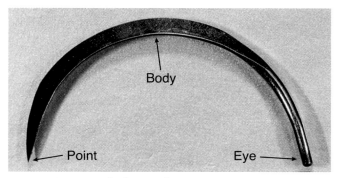

FIGURE 4-7 Parts of a free needle.

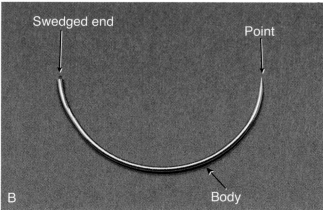

FIGURE 4-6 Parts of a suture needle: A) straight and B) curved.

The swedged end (see Fig. 4-6) is where the suture is attached. This is done by the manufacturer. Most sutures are made this way. There are two common types of swedged ends: a controlled release or "pop off." Once the surgeon has placed the suture, he or she can give the needle a tug and it "pops off," leaving only the needle in the needle holder. The other type is permanently swedged to the needle, requiring that the needle be cut off of the suture.

The free needle (see Fig. 4-7) does not have a suture attached. This needle has an eye, like a sewing needle, through which a suture can be threaded.

There are several different types of suture needle points. Each point was designed with a specific purpose in mind. The following describe the features and general uses for each type of needle point.

Name: conventional cutting needle
Features: three cutting edges; the third one is located on the inside concave curvature of the needle
Use: closes skin or secures drains

Name: reverse cutting needle
Features: three cutting edges; the third one is located on the outer convex curvature of the needle
Use: designed for use on tough tissue (muscle, skin or fascia)

Name: heavy body reverse cutting needle
Features: heavy needle body; ½ circle curvature
Use: closes muscle, fascia, bone, skin and cartilage

Name: premium X-cutting needle
Features: four-sided plastic surgery cutting edge
Use: closes cuticle and subcuticle

Name: spatula (side cutting) needle

Features: flat on top and bottom; eliminates the tissue cutout of a cutting point

Use: designed for use in ophthalmic procedures

Name: taper needle

Features: pierces and spreads tissue without cutting it; used in easily penetrated tissue; very common needle point

Use: can be used on most tissues inside the body cavity

Name: taper cut (trocar point) needle

Features: combines the features of a reverse cutting point and taper point

Use: sutures dense, fibrous tissue

Name: blunt needle

Features: dissects the tissue rather than cutting it

Use: sutures friable tissue such as liver and kidney

Name: endoscopic needle

Features: taper point

Use: used in laparoscopic procedures

(Sources of information: *Ethicon Wound Closure Manual* (2004); www.syneture.com; www.Alcon.com.)

WATCH OUT!

Suture Needle Safety

When handling suture needles, several safety precautions must be taken to minimize the risk of needlestick injury to oneself or others.

- Load the suture needle directly onto the needle holder; do not pick it up with your fingers to load it.

- When possible, load needles just before use to avoid open needles on the back table or Mayo stand.

- Put your needles and needle holders in the same place on your back table or Mayo stand each time you set up and during surgery. By placing them in the same place every time, you know where they are and are less apt accidently to get stuck when you reach for other instruments.

- Know where your needles are at all times. Know the location of needles on the surgical field, your Mayo stand and back table. If the surgeon says "needle back" or "needle down," look to see where he or she placed it (especially if your institution does not use a neutral zone).

- Use a neutral zone for passing and receiving suture needles. A neutral zone is a designated area when the scrubbed person places the loaded needle holder. The surgeon (or assistant) picks up the loaded needle holder from the designated area. When the surgeon or assistant is done with the suture, he or she places the used needle and needle holder back in the neutral zone. The scrubbed person takes the used needle and holder back from the neutral zone; there is no hand-to-hand passing. This helps avoid the chance of being stuck during hand-to-hand passing. *Note:* Not all facilities currently use the neutral zone; check your institution's policies and procedures.

- Place all used needles in a puncture-proof foam or magnetic needle counter (Accu-Count or other device). Placing each used needle in a counter keeps them in one place (not all over your back table), makes it easier to count needles and lessens the likelihood of being stuck by a stray needle.

- At the end of the case, dispose of all needles and the needle counter (AccuCount) in a puncture-proof biohazard waste box.

INDIVIDUAL SUTURE NEEDLES

There are two major manufacturers of suture material: Ethicon and Syneture (US Suture and Davis and Geck). The suture needles described in this section contain the name the manufacturer gave the needle as well as comparable needles (where applicable) made by the other manufacturer.

Name: ⅜ cutting needle
Alias: none
Use: sutures skin
Features: conventional cutting point
Additional Information: ⅜ circle shape

Name: LH needle (Ethicon)
Alias: large ½ (circle) needle
Use: passes through dense or thick dermal tissue
Features: cutting point
Additional Information: ½ circle shape

Name: Keith needle (Ethicon)

Alias: straight needle; KS needle

Comparable needle: SC-2 (Syneture)

Use: closes skin of abdominal wounds

Features: cutting point

Additional Information: available in varying lengths and sizes

Name: T needle

Alias: taper needle

Use: passes sutures through large areas or wounds

Features: taper point

Additional Information: ½ circle shape; available in a variety of sizes

Name: G needle (Ethicon)

Alias: Grieshaber ⅜ (circle) needle

Comparable needle: HE (Syneture)

Use: closes skin

Features: micropoint cutting point

Additional Information: ⅜ circle shape

Name: GS needle (Ethicon)

Alias: Grieshaber spatula

Use: sutures easily penetrated tissue (e.g., abdominal viscera and peritoneum)

Features: spatula point; pierces and spreads tissue without cutting

Additional Information: ½ circle shape

Name: LR needle (Ethicon)

Alias: larger retention needle

Comparable needle: GS-18 (Syneture)

Use: inserts retention sutures

Features: large, heavy needle for penetrating multiple layers of tissue; cutting point

Additional Information: bolsters may be used if the surgeon is placing retention sutures

Name: Martin uterine needle

Alias: none

Use: installs sutures through uterine or other heavier tissue

Features: cutting edge; closed eye; free needle (does not come with suture attached)

Additional Information: ½ circle shape

Name: V tapercut needle (Ethicon)

Alias: tapercut surgical needle

Comparable needle: KV (Syneture)

Use: puts sutures in dense, thick tissue

Features: three cutting edges extend from the point (known as a *trocar point*); more uniform cutting

Additional Information: comes in a variety of circle types (½ circle, ⅜ circle, etc) and sizes

Name: CTX needle (Ethicon)

Alias: circle taper extra large needle

Comparable needle: GS-25 (Syneture)

Use: installs sutures in easily penetrated tissue

Features: pierces and spreads tissue without cutting

Additional Information: ½ circle shape; used in large areas or on large viscera

Name: PC needle (Ethicon)

Alias: precision cosmetic needle

Comparable needle: PC-10 (Syneture)

Use: closes skin in cosmetic surgery

Features: fine point; conventional cutting point

Additional Information: narrow needle body taper

Name: PS needle (Ethicon)

Alias: plastic surgery needle

Comparable needle: P (Syneture)

Use: approximates tissue in plastic surgery

Features: fine point; reverse cutting point

Additional Information: ⅜ circle shape; available in a variety of sizes

Name: SH needle (Ethicon)
Alias: small half (circle) needle
Comparable needle: CV-24, CV-25 (Syneture)
Use: sutures easily penetrated tissue
Features: taper point
Additional Information: ½ circle shape; available in a variety of sizes

Name: FS needle (Ethicon)
Alias: for skin needle
Comparable needle: C (Syneture)
Use: closes skin; sutures drains in place
Features: reverse cutting point
Additional Information: ⅜ circle shape; available in a variety of sizes

Name: CT needle (Ethicon)
Alias: circle taper needle
Comparable needle: GS-24 (Syneture)
Use: sutures easily penetrated tissue (e.g., abdominal viscera and peritoneum)
Features: taper point; available on some sutures as a controlled-release ("pop-off") needle
Additional Information: ½ circle shape; available in a variety of sizes

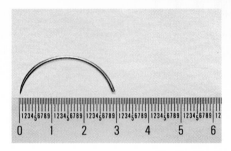

Name: RB needle (Ethicon)
Alias: renal (artery) bypass needle
Comparable needle: CV, CVF (Syneture)
Use: sutures tissue in urological procedures
Features: taper tip
Additional Information: ⅝ circle shape

Name: CP needle (Ethicon)
Alias: cutting point needle
Comparable needle: GS-10, GS-11, GS-12 (Syneture)
Use: approximates skin
Features: cutting point
Additional Information: ⅜ circle shape; available in a variety of sizes

Name: CE needle (Ethicon)
Alias: cutting edge needle
Use: approximates skin; sutures dense, thick tissue
Features: cutting point
Additional Information: ½ circle shape; available in a variety of sizes

Name: Davis Tonsil needle
Alias: none
Use: installs sutures in the throat and mouth
Features: taper point; closed eye; free needle (does not come with suture attached)
Additional Information: ½ circle shape

Name: Mayo Catgut needle
Alias: none
Use: works for general tissue approximation (not for use on heavy tissue)
Features: taper point; closed eye; free needle (does not come with suture attached)
Additional Information: ½ circle shape

Name: Ferguson needle
Alias: none
Use: taper point (round body)
Features: delicate tissue approximation; free needle (does not come with suture attached)
Additional Information: ½ circle shape

Name: S needle (Ethicon)
Alias: spatula needle
Comparable needle: SS (Syneture)
Use: sutures delicate tissue; ophthalmic surgery
Features: flat on top and bottom with side cutting edges to separate or split through thin layers of tissue (spatula point)
Additional Information: available in a variety of sizes

Name: MO needle (Ethicon)

Alias: Mayo needle

Comparable needle: HGS (Syneture)

Use: sutures dense tissue in gynecological surgery, hernia repair and general tissue closure

Features: taper point with a heavier, more flat body

Additional Information: ½ circle shape; available in a variety of sizes

Name: OS needle (Ethicon)

Alias: orthopedic surgery needle

Comparable needle: HOS (Syneture)

Use: sutures heavy tissue (ligaments, tendons)

Features: reverse cutting tip

Additional Information: ½ circle shape; available in a variety of sizes

Name: UR needle (Ethicon)

Alias: urology needle

Comparable needle: GU (Syneture)

Use: sutures around or under structures during urology procedures

Features: taper point

Additional Information: ⅝ circle shape; available in a variety of sizes

Name: SBE needle (Ethicon)

Alias: slim blade needle

Use: sutures delicate structures

Features: taper point needle

Additional Information: ½ circle shape; taper point pierces and spreads tissue without cutting it

Name: HOS needle (Syneture)

Alias: heavy orthopedic surgery needle

Comparable needle: OS (Ethicon)

Use: approximates heavy soft tissue (e.g., meniscal repair)

Features: reverse cutting point

Additional Information: ½ circle shape

Name: BB needle (Ethicon)
Alias: blue baby needle
Comparable needle: CV, CVF (Syneture)
Use: used in cardiovascular surgery
Features: taper point
Additional Information: ⅜ circle shape

Name: TG needle (Ethicon)
Alias: transverse ground needle
Comparable needle: SE (Syneture)
Use: used in ophthalmic procedures
Features: flat on top and bottom with side cutting edges to separate or split through thin layers of tissue (spatula point)
Additional Information: ⅜ circle shape

Name: C needle (Ethicon)
Alias: cardiovascular needle
Comparable needle: CV, CVF (Syneture)
Use: used in cardiovascular surgery
Features: taper point
Additional Information: ½ circle shape

Name: BV needle (Ethicon)
Alias: blood vessel needle
Comparable needle: MV, MVK (Syneture)
Use: sutures fine blood vessels
Features: taper point
Additional Information: ⅜ circle shape; usually comes as a double-armed suture (two needles: one on each end of the suture)

Name: MH needle (Ethicon)
Alias: medium ½ (circle) needle
Comparable needle: CV-300, V-26 (Syneture)
Use: used for general tissue approximation
Features: taper point
Additional Information: ½ circle shape

Name: TF needle (Ethicon)

Alias: tetralogy of Fallot needle

Comparable needle: CV-17, CV-18, CV-21

Use: used in pediatric cardiac repair

Features: taper point; very delicate needle

Additional Information: ½ circle shape; very delicate needle, must be handled with a micro-surgery needle holder

Name: X needle (Ethicon)

Alias: exodontal needle

Comparable needle: C-23 (Syneture)

Use: used for dental surgery

Features: reverse cutting point

Additional Information: ½ circle shape

Name: BP needle (Ethicon)

Alias: blunt point needle

Comparable needle: BGS-28 (Syneture)

Use: used to perform blunt dissection of friable tissue (e.g., liver, kidney, cervix, intestine, spleen)

Features: blunt taper point

Additional Information: ½ circle shape; available in a variety of sizes

Name: J needle (Ethicon)

Alias: conjunctive needle

Comparable needle: C-22, C-26 (Syneture)

Use: used in ophthalmic procedures; sutures delicate tissue

Features: reverse cutting tip

Additional Information: ½ circle shape; available in a variety of sizes

Name: VAS needle

Alias: vas deferens needle

Use: anastomoses the vas deferens during vasovasostomy; microsurgery

Features: micropoint (smooth surface, very sharp point)

Additional Information: very delicate needle, must be handled with a microsurgery needle holder

Name: P needle (Syneture)
Alias: plastic needle
Comparable needle: P (Ethicon)
Use: used in cosmetic surgery
Features: reverse cutting point
Additional Information: ⅜ circle shape; available in a variety of sizes

Name: FSL needle (Ethicon)
Alias: for skin large needle
Comparable needle: C-17 (Syneture)
Use: closes skin in large wounds
Features: reverse cutting point
Additional Information: ⅜ circle shape; available in a variety of sizes

Name: STC needle
Alias: straight cutting needle
Use: used in ophthalmic procedures; microsurgery procedures
Features: side cutting spatula tip; needle is straight
Additional Information: available in a variety of lengths

Name: TT needle (Gore Medical)
Alias: none
Use: used in cardiac or vascular surgery
Features: taper point
Additional Information: ⅜ circle shape; available in a variety of sizes; usually comes on a double armed Gore-Tex suture (two needles: one on each end of the suture)

Name: PH needle (Gore Medical)
Alias: none
Use: used in cardiac or vascular surgery
Features: piercing point
Additional Information: ½ circle shape; available in a variety of sizes; usually comes on a double-armed Gore-Tex suture (two needles: one on each end of the suture)

Name: HE needle (Syneture)

Alias: none

Comparable needle: G (Ethicon)

Use: used for general tissue approximation

Features: reverse cutting point

Additional Information: ⅜ circle shape

Name: HGS needle (Syneture)

Alias: heavy Grieshaber

Comparable needle: MO (Ethicon)

Use: sutures heavy tissue

Features: taper point

Additional Information: ½ circle shape; available in a variety of sizes

Name: Mayo Intestinal needle

Alias: none

Use: sutures bowel; used in general tissue approximation

Features: taper point; closed eye

Additional Information: free needle (does not come with suture attached)

 Surgical Session Review

1) The surgeon is finishing cardiac bypass surgery and is ready to close the sternum. Which suture is she most likely to use?
a. nylon
b. Prolene
c. stainless steel
d. Monocryl

2) The surgeon wishes to put retention sutures into a large midline abdominal wound. Which suture would be the most appropriate for you to have ready?
a. 4-0 nylon
b. 5 Ethibond
c. 5-0 Prolene
d. 5-0 Vicryl

3) Used needles and sharps should be placed in a(n) _____ on the field.
a. AccuCheck
b. AccuCount
c. paper trash bag
d. kidney basin

4) _____ is a liquid, topical skin adhesive.
a. Dermabond
b. DuraPrep
c. Duralon
d. Dermabrade

5) Which of the following is made of nylon fiber?
   a. Monocryl
   b. Panacryl
   c. Vicryl
   d. Ethilon

6) One of the following sutures does NOT have memory, thus eliminating the need to give it a gentle tug prior to handing it to the surgeon. Which suture does NOT have memory?
   a. Maxon
   b. Prolene
   c. Chromic
   d. Vicryl

7) During eye surgery, which of the following sutures would most likely be used?
   a. 4 Ethilon
   b. 2 Ethilon
   c. 2-0 Ethilon
   d. 9-0 Ethilon

8) All but one of the following are non-absorbable sutures. Which one is the absorbable suture?
   a. stainless steel
   b. Ethilon
   c. Vicryl
   d. Prolene

9) Another name for a straight needle is a(n) _____ needle.
   a. Kevin
   b. Keith
   c. LH
   d. CT

10) The "PS" in PS needle stands for:
   a. pointed straight
   b. plain suture
   c. plastic surgery
   d. pointed suture

11) The surgeon requests a taper point needle. Which of the following would be appropriate to hand him?
   a. CP needle
   b. CT needle
   c. CE needle
   d. OS needle

12) An RB needle is usually used during what type of procedures?
   a. cardiovascular
   b. gynecological
   c. urological
   d. obstetrical

13) An MH needle has a _____ circle shape.
   a. ¼
   b. ⅜
   c. ½
   d. ⅝

14) The needle designed specifically for suturing in the throat (tonsils) is a:
   a. Davis
   b. Ferguson
   c. Martin
   d. Mayo Catgut

15) The S needle has a _____ point.
   a. cutting
   b. taper
   c. taper point
   d. spatula

16) What type of needle would most likely be used to place retention sutures into a large abdominal wound?
   a. PC
   b. LR
   c. Martin
   d. PS

17) Which of these suture sizes is the heaviest (thickest)?
   1. 3
   2. 0
   3. 2-0
   4. 3-0

18) Gore-Tex suture is:
   a. monofilament
   b. multifilament
   c. braided
   d. polyfilament

19) All of the following statements about sharps safety are true *except:*
   a. use a neutral zone when passing sharps
   b. know where your needles and sharps are located at all times
   c. load needles as far in advance of use as possible
   d. at the end of the case, dispose of all needles in a puncture-proof container

20) A needle without a suture attached is called a(n) _____ needle.
   a. swedged
   b. free
   c. orphaned
   d. solo

CHAPTER 5

Endoscopic Equipment

ENDOSCOPIC SURGERY

The root word *endo* means "within." The suffix *scopy* means "to view with an instrument." The term *endoscopy* means "using an instrument to view within (a body cavity)." Endoscopy is a general term referring to any procedure that uses a scope to view inside a body cavity, but there are several terms that are used to be more specific about which area is being viewed:

- *Anoscopy:* Viewing inside the anus
- *Arthroscopy:* Viewing inside a joint
- *Bronchoscopy:* Viewing inside the lungs (bronchus)
- *Colonoscopy:* Viewing inside the colon
- *Colposcopy:* Viewing inside the vagina and cervix
- *Cystoscopy:* Viewing inside the bladder
- *Duodenoscopy:* Viewing inside the duodenum
- *Esophagoscopy:* Viewing inside the esophagus
- *Esophagogastroduodenoscopy (EGD):* Viewing inside the esophagus, stomach and duodenum
- *Fluoroscopy:* Viewing inside organs or tissues using x-ray
- *Gastroscopy:* Viewing inside the stomach
- *Hepatoscopy:* Viewing the liver
- *Hysteroscopy:* Viewing inside the uterus
- *Laparoscopy:* Viewing inside the abdominal and pelvic cavities
- *Laryngoscopy:* Viewing inside the larynx
- *Meatoscopy:* Viewing inside the urinary meatus
- *Mediastinoscopy:* Viewing inside the mediastinum (mediastinal space)
- *Pelvioscopy (pelvoscopy):* Viewing inside the pelvis
- *Pharyngoscopy:* Viewing inside the throat
- *Rhinoscopy:* Viewing inside the nose
- *Sigmoidoscopy:* Viewing inside the sigmoid colon
- *Thoracoscopy (pleuroscopy):* Viewing inside the chest (thorax)
- *Tracheoscopy:* Viewing inside the trachea
- *Ureteroscopy:* Viewing inside the ureter
- *Urethroscopy:* Viewing inside the urethra

When a surgical procedure is performed using a scope and very small incisions (known as *stab wound* incisions), it is referred to as *minimally invasive surgery.* Minimally invasive surgery came onto the surgical scene in the 1980s and revolutionized the way surgery is performed. Today, more and more procedures (including gastric bypass and coronary bypass surgeries) are being performed using minimally invasive techniques.

There are several advantages to minimally invasive surgery, including smaller incisions (less scarring and less pain), reduced length of hospital stay, reduced time recovering at home and less time out of work. The actual time it takes to perform a minimally invasive procedure in the operating room (OR) is not shorter than an open procedure, but the advantages of less pain and disability for the patient as well as less tissue trauma are reasons to perform the procedure endoscopically.

It must be stated that not every procedure can or should be performed endoscopically. Some procedures still must be performed as open procedures (e.g., in the presence of a large, infected gallbladder). Often, it is not known until the surgery has begun and the surgeon has had a chance to look inside whether or not the surgery can be safely performed endoscopically. For this reason, every endoscopic case should be set up with the ability to convert to an open case quickly and easily. Most of the time, this means setting up two sets of instruments on the back table: endoscopic instruments and a traditional stringer of instruments to be used for an open case.

Every minimally invasive procedure requires certain basic equipment: a video viewing system (TV system), a recording system (still pictures, videotape or DVD) and a light source for the camera. Procedures involving the abdomen and pelvis require a gas (carbon dioxide) insufflating system. Procedures involving the joints or urinary system require a constant fluid irrigation system. This is usually normal saline, but for some urinary procedures, glycine is used.

The following sections of this chapter cover video towers (including basic troubleshooting), cameras, scopes and equipment (including care and cleaning) and some specifics for arthroscopic, flexible and rigid scopes.

VIDEO TOWERS

Minimally invasive procedures require the surgeon to be able to view inside the body cavity where he or she is working. This is done using a camera with the image projected up onto a video system (usually a TV system of some sort).

Although the types of video systems vary from institution to institution, the requirement is the same; scrubbed personnel must be able to view clearly and easily what is going on inside the operative field. The simplest way to accomplish this is to have two TV towers, one on each side of the patient, toward the head of the bed so that personnel on both sides of the operative field are looking directly at a monitor (Fig. 5-1).

FIGURE 5-1 Two video towers.

FIGURE 5-2 Light source box.

This set up may vary depending on the procedure and the surgeon as some procedures may require the use of only one tower at the foot of the bed or, in the case of cystoscopy, there may be one monitor mounted on a moveable arm directly over the patient. In any case, the set up needs to meet the requirement of clear and easy viewing by scrubbed personnel.

In addition to the monitor or TV screen, there needs to be a device for recording pictures. The device can be as simple as a printer for still photographs or as advanced as a DVD recording system. The type of system used depends on the institution and the equipment available.

The third basic component of the system is the light source for the camera (see Fig. 5-2). The type of light source used is dependent on the camera system being used. It is the

responsibility of the OR team assigned to the case to ensure that the camera being used is compatible with the light source.

The last component is the source of insufflation. For procedures of the abdomen and pelvis, insufflation is accomplished using carbon dioxide gas. The gas pressure and rate of gas flow into the abdominal cavity are regulated through the use of an insufflator (see Fig. 5-3). The settings on the insufflator vary according to the surgeon and procedure, but a safe flow of gas (start low and then increase as needed) should be used until a pressure of around 15 mm Hg (varies from 12 to 18 mm Hg) is achieved.

Remember: Always check the gas level in your carbon dioxide tank before the start of a case. Change the tank if the gas is low or empty. Do not start a procedure with a tank that does not have sufficient gas to complete the case.

When doing endoscopic procedures of the joints or bladder, you will be using fluid rather than gas to expand the cavity for visualization. In most cases, this requires the use of a fluid pump, although some simple urologic procedures can be done using a gravity-fed bag (see Fig. 5-4). Although different pumps are used for arthroscopic procedures versus urology procedures, the principles are the same; the fluid needs to be pumped into and drained out of the cavity continuously throughout the entire procedure. It is imperative that the circulator (or whoever is in charge of the fluids) makes sure that bags are replaced as soon as they get low; it is not OK for the fluid to run dry. Some pumps have a low fluid warning alarm to alert personnel when the bag is getting low, but do not rely

---

WATCH OUT! **Recording of Pictures**

- Recording surgery is dictated by institutional policies and procedures. Know your institution's policies surrounding the recording of procedures *prior* to starting any case in which pictures or video will be shot.

- Usually, for still pictures that are going to be placed in the medical record, a special release is not required because these pictures are part of the medical record and not likely to be viewed by others.

- For video recording that is going to be used for educational purposes, a special release may need to be signed by the patient before surgery. Be sure to check your institution's policy!

WATCH OUT! **Potential Fire Hazard**

- *Caution:* The light source is a source of heat and could be a potential fire hazard!

- When the camera is not in use and is outside the body, place it in *standby* mode.

- A camera with its light source *not* in standby mode should *never* be placed on the drapes as it could overheat and cause a fire.

FIGURE 5–3 Insufflator box.

FIGURE 5–5 Two video towers at the head of the bed.

FIGURE 5–4 Fluid pump.

FIGURE 5–6 One video tower at bottom of bed.

on the alarm. You must be vigilant, watch the fluid level in the bags and replace them before they run dry.

Video Tower Set Up

As stated earlier, there are a couple of variations of video tower arrangements, depending on the procedure being done and surgeon preference. The most common set up for general laparoscopic procedures is two video monitors, one on each side of the bed, about the level of the patient's shoulders (see Fig. 5-5). This allows the operative field to be viewed by scrubbed personnel standing on either side of the patient. This type of set up requires two monitors: a primary monitor and a secondary monitor. The primary monitor is the one attached

to the camera box and receives the picture by direct input. The secondary monitor is attached to the primary monitor with a video cable. The towers are not sterile; make sure they are placed at least 12 to 18 inches away from the draped patient.

The second arrangement requires the use of one video tower. This tower may be placed at the foot of the bed or to one side at the head of the bed by the patient's shoulder (see Fig. 5-6). The tower is not sterile; make sure it is at least 12 to 18 inches away from the draped patient. This type of set up is most commonly used for some gynecological and cystoscopic procedures.

All video towers and equipment *must* be checked by the staff assigned to the procedure prior to bringing the patient into the OR. Equipment must be plugged in, turned on and checked to make sure it is functioning properly. If it is not functioning properly and cannot be easily fixed (see Troubleshooting Tips), it must be removed from the room and another piece of equipment brought in and tested.

At the end of the case, all video towers and equipment should be wiped down with disinfectant, according to your institution's policy, before leaving the room or being used for a subsequent procedure.

ENDOSCOPIC CAMERAS

The invention of cameras that fit onto the eyepiece of rigid endoscopes has revolutionized surgery. The surgeon is no longer the only one able to visualize the operative field; cameras enable the entire surgical team to watch the procedure and anticipate what might be needed next. In some cases (depending on the institution), a scrub person operates the camera, freeing up both of the surgeon's hands to perform the procedure. Before the invention of endoscopic cameras, the surgeon would have to use one hand to hold the scope so that he or she could look through the eyepiece.

The camera set up consists of a camera head with a cord and a coupler (see Fig. 5-7). In some newer models, the camera and coupler are one piece. The camera cord attaches to a video box that is attached to the video monitor (TV screen) to allow the entire team to view the procedure. Procedures

FIGURE 5–7 A) Camera components. B) Assembled camera.

Troubleshooting Tips

Video equipment and towers are mechanical machines and may, from time to time, not work properly. Here are some simple troubleshooting tips. Always refer to manufacturer's instructions for more in-depth advice.

PROBLEM	WHAT TO LOOK AT
I turn on the video monitor but do not get color bars. (On some monitors, the presence of vertical color bars tells you the monitor is properly hooked up and working.)	■ Check to make sure the cables are hooked into the proper connections in the back of the monitor (especially if you have color bars on the primary monitor but not the secondary one). ■ Make sure *all* components of the system are powered on. (Some monitors will not work even if it is the printer that is not turned on.)
The picture is blurred or streaked.	■ Check the lenses of the scope and camera; they may be dirty or need defogging.
The color on the monitor screen is not accurate.	■ The camera may need to be re-white balanced; white balance the camera again.
The monitor screen is dark; there is nothing on it.	■ Make sure the monitor is plugged in and turned on (check this first). ■ Check cables to make sure they are intact and hooked into the proper connections. ■ Check to make sure the power box is not overloaded with too many devices plugged into it. ■ Check the fuses. ■ Check the connection to the printer to make sure it is properly connected.
The still pictures did not print (or are of poor quality).	■ Make sure to print the pictures *before* turning off the printer at the end of the case. ■ The printer is out of paper. ■ The paper is in upside down. ■ The cartridge is low or out of ink or toner.
The pictures are blurred when printed.	■ The camera or scope lens is dirty or fogged up. ■ There was movement by the person operating the camera during picture taking.

can be documented on video or in still photographs. The newer models have digital and HDTV picture recording for better quality and sharper resolution and some allow recording onto DVD rather than tape.

The camera head and cord are attached to the endoscope using a coupler. The camera head screws onto the coupler, and the endoscope is attached to the other end using a built-in clamp. The clamp opens to allow you to slip the scope eyepiece into it and then closes around it to hold the eyepiece snuggly in place. After attaching the camera and scope to the coupler, check to make sure the connections are tight and neither the camera nor scope is wobbly.

At the end of the case, the camera, cord and coupler should be cleaned and sterilized according to manufacturer's instructions. *Read the instructions carefully prior to autoclaving any camera, coupler or cord.* Not all models are able to be autoclaved; doing so will result in severe damage (lens breakage, melting of casing, fiberoptic damage).

Care of Endoscopic Cameras

- Attach the camera and turn it on prior to surgery to make sure it works. If the light cable is fiberoptic, check it. If the cable contains dark areas where you cannot see light coming through, replace the cable as these dark areas can be indicative of broken fibers.
- *Never* place cameras at the bottom of an instrument tray. The weight of the other instruments could damage the camera.
- When you are setting up your table, never place anything else on top of the camera. Cameras are very delicate and another instrument or piece of equipment could easily damage it.
- When coiling the camera cord, never coil it tighter than a soda can diameter. Coiling the cord too tight can result in damage and breakage of the fiberoptic fibers.
- Follow manufacturer's instructions for cleaning and sterilizing cameras, cords and couplers. After cleaning, inspect the components for cleanliness and possible damage.
- Never use anything abrasive to clean the camera, lens or components.

RIGID SCOPE COMPONENTS

Although the scope (sometimes referred to as a *telescope*) is a single instrument, it is composed of several components: the eyepiece (contains the proximal or ocular lens), the light attachment, the shaft and the distal (or objective) lens.

The proximal end of the scope contains the eyepiece or ocular lens. In older models of scopes, the proximal end is made for direct viewing into the cavity with your eye. These types of scopes allowed only the surgeon to view the surgical field. In most modern scopes, the proximal end is where the camera attaches to the scope to allow for projection of the

image onto the screen, enabling all members of the surgical team to view the operative field.

The light attachment sticks up at a 90-degree angle near the eyepiece at the proximal end of the scope. This is where the light cord (usually a fiberoptic cable) attaches to the scope. The other end of the light cord is passed off to the circulator and attached into the light source box.

The shaft of the scope is the long, thin part of the instrument that is inserted through the trocar into the body cavity. The shaft is very delicate and must be handled with care as it is easily damaged or bent and expensive to repair (see Care of Rigid Endoscopes, later in this section). Shaft diameters vary from 1.9 mm to 10 mm, with 5 mm and 10 mm being the ones most commonly used.

The distal or objective lens is at the end of the shaft. It is used to view and magnify the organs or tissues. Scopes are available with a variety of angles of objective lenses to allow for viewing around structures. The most common objective lenses are the 0 degree (also known as the *forward* or *straight-on*), 30 degree (*forward-oblique*), 45 degree and 70 degree.

Objective lenses on the scopes become distorted or fog up due to blood, fluid or debris. It is important that the scrub personnel have lens defogger available during surgery to clean the objective lens. If the picture becomes unsatisfactory, the scope should be removed from the body cavity, the lens gently wiped clean, the defogger applied and the scope reinserted through the trocar. If the picture remains unsatisfactory, the camera may need to be removed from the eyepiece and the camera lenses and eyepiece (ocular lens) cleaned.

Care of Rigid Endoscopes

- Never pick up and hold scopes by the distal end. The weight of the eyepiece could easily bend the shaft.
- Scrubbed personnel must look through the eyepiece before attaching the camera before surgery. If what he or she sees is distorted or cloudy, the eyepiece and objective lens must be cleaned. If cleaning does not clear up the problem, get another scope because one (or both) of the lenses may be damaged and need repair or replacement.
- Prior to surgery, check the scope shaft for damage, dents or bends. If the scope is damaged, get another one.
- Attach the camera and turn it on prior to surgery to make sure it works. If the light cable is fiberoptic, check it. If the cable contains dark areas where you cannot see light coming through, replace the cable as these dark areas can be indicative of broken fibers.
- *Never* place scopes at the bottom of an instrument tray. The weight of the other instruments could bend or damage the scope. Place the scope in the storage case that it comes in.
- When not in use, set the scope on a flat surface to avoid accidental flexion and damage.
- When you are setting up your table, never place anything else on top of the scope. Scopes are very

delicate, and another instrument or piece of equipment could easily damage it.

- When handing the scope to the surgeon or using the scope during a procedure, support the shaft of the scope with one hand to avoid overflexion and possible damage.

- When coiling the light cord, never coil it tighter than a soda can diameter. Coiling the cord too tight can result in damage and breakage of the fiberoptic fibers.

- Follow manufacturer's instructions for cleaning and sterilizing scopes. Make sure all lumens and valves are cleaned and rinsed thoroughly prior to sterilization. After cleaning, inspect the scope for cleanliness and possible damage.

(Some material adapted from Karl Storz website.)

CYSTOSCOPY/URETEROSCOPY EQUIPMENT

Cystoscopy means viewing into the bladder, although this procedure is done most of the time for more than just "viewing." This procedure can be done for diagnostic purposes (e.g., to find the source of blood in the urine), as part of the treatment of a urological condition (e.g., to remove or resect bladder tumors, remove kidney stones or resect the prostate) or for ureteral stent insertion. Cystoscopy can also be done at the end of another procedure to check for inadvertent damage to the bladder.

The cystoscope (also known as a *cystourethroscope*) has several pieces that the scrub person needs to assemble (see Fig. 5-8). The *sheath* is the hollow tube that allows for the passage of instruments during the procedure and allows for suction and irrigation. The main (large) channel in the center of the sheath is where the *telescope* is inserted. The side channels allow accessory instruments to be used, such as biopsy forceps or graspers. The *obturator* is a rod with a round, blunt tip. The obturator is inserted into the main channel of the sheath and used just during the insertion of the scope. The obturator helps protect urethral tissue from damage. Once the sheath is inserted through the

FIGURE 5-8 Cystoscopy equipment.

- Read the manufacturer's instructions for cleaning and sterilizing the cystoscope. Some cystoscopes and attachments are able to be autoclaved (steam sterilized) and some are not. Make sure you know if your scope, camera, cords and so on can be autoclaved prior to the sterilization process.

- Handle the scope by the *middle* of the shaft. Do not handle it by the ends or it could bend.

- Do not place anything on top of the scope. Do not place it at the bottom of a pan of instruments. For transport, place it in the storage container that it came in.

- Do not the coil cord too tightly; this could damage or break the fiberoptic bundles.

- When setting up your sterile field prior to the case, check all scopes and accessories for damage (e.g., bending, cracks in the cord casing). Put the scope together and make sure you have all the pieces (e.g., sheath, telescope, obturator, bridge and instruments). Make sure all instruments are functioning properly.

- When cleaning and sterilizing the cystoscopes after use, make sure all stopcocks are open.

urethra, the obturator is removed and the telescope inserted. Like all endoscopes, the telescope portion of the cystoscope needs a light cable hooked to it that is attached to a light source. Depending on what procedure is being performed, a *bridge* may need to be attached to the scope to allow for the use of accessory instruments.

Cystoscopes vary in the degree of the angle of the scope's tip. The most common cystoscopes used are 0 degrees, 30 degrees and 70 degrees. Make sure you have the correct scope for the procedure and that any back-up scopes that may be needed are available.

Continuous irrigation is necessary for cystoscopic procedures. The solution can be instilled using gravity, although some procedures or institutions may require the use of a pump. Suction with a large volume capacity (e.g., Neptune or large suction carousel) is necessary to handle the continuous outflow of fluid. Normal saline is the irrigation fluid most commonly used for procedures not requiring the use of electrocautery. If the use of electrocautery is anticipated, a *nonelectrolytic* solution, such as 3% sorbitol or glycine, is used. *Nonelectrolytic* means that the fluid is unable to transmit or disperse electricity from the electrode tip. It is the responsibility of the circulator to make sure that the fluid does not run out during the procedure; therefore, he or she must monitor the fluid bags and change them as needed (see Fig. 5-9).

Many institutions have a special room dedicated to cystoscopic procedures. This room is equipped with a table that allows for fluoroscopic imaging during the procedure (see Fig. 5-10). Lithotomy (legs up in stirrups) is the position of choice for many cystoscopic procedures; therefore, the cystoscopy table is able to have stirrups attached to it.

Some procedures require the use of laser or fluoroscopy intraoperatively. Make sure to turn on the fluoroscopy machine or laser before bringing the patient into the room to make

FIGURE 5–9 Continuous irrigation set up.

FIGURE 5–10 Cystoscopy table.

FIGURE 5–11 Ureteroscope.

done for treatment of kidney stones, but it can be diagnostic as well. For the treatment of kidney stones, the urologist inserts the ureteroscope up into the ureter until he or she finds the stone(s). Then, depending on the size and location of the stone(s), the urologist may use a special instrument called a *stone retrieval basket* (see Fig. 5-12B) to snare each stone and remove it or may opt to insert a laser fiber (see Fig. 5-12A) and shatter each stone using laser energy.

FIGURE 5–12 A) Laser fiber. B) Stone retrieval basket.

sure the machine is functioning properly. If the use of fluoroscopy is anticipated, make sure there are lead aprons available for all staff to wear (including thyroid shields). If the use of laser is anticipated, make sure that all safety equipment is available and all laser safety precautions are followed (see Chapter 6 for more on laser safety).

Ureteroscopy

A ureteroscope is a very long, thin scope designed to be inserted into the urethra, to go through the bladder and to move into the ureter (see Fig. 5-11). Most often this procedure is

Ureteroscopes are available in rigid, semi-rigid and flexible models. Which type is used depends on surgeon preference and the location of the stone.

As with all scopes, take care when handling the ureteroscope. It is longer than traditional cystoscopes; therefore, the scrub person must always be aware of the location of the tip of the scope to avoid inadvertent contamination or damage from the tip hitting against something. Handle the scope with two hands, supporting it in the middle and at the eyepiece end to avoid bending the shaft.

Positioning for ureteroscopy is the same as for cystoscopy; the patient is placed in the lithotomy position on the cystoscopy table.

RIGID ENT/THORACIC SCOPES

Rigid Laryngoscopes for Direct Laryngoscopy

Rigid laryngoscopes are used to see directly within the throat, usually for one of the following purposes:

- Biopsy throat lesions.
- Diagnose causes of hoarse voice, weak voice or no voice.
- Identify unknown cause of chronic sore throat.
- Evaluate difficulty swallowing.
- See injuries or obstructions in the throat (e.g., tumors, masses or strictures).
- Remove foreign bodies from the throat.
- Remove vocal cord polyps.
- Perform laser treatments on throat lesions.

The rigid laryngoscope set up consists of the scope, the light cord or light fibers and a light source box (see Fig. 5-13). Some direct laryngoscopy set ups attach to a camera, enabling the entire surgical team to view the throat on a monitor.

The surgeon requires suction and may need flexible biopsy forceps, cup forceps or graspers, depending on the procedure being performed. If the patient is undergoing a microlaryngoscopy, a suspension device is placed on the patient's chest to hold the rigid laryngoscope, leaving the surgeon's hands free to operate the microscope and instruments. Before the insertion of a rigid laryngoscope, a mouth guard is placed over the patient's upper teeth to protect them from damage.

Patient positioning varies according to institution or surgeon preference, but generally the patient is placed supine with a shoulder roll and doughnut headrest.

Rigid Bronchoscopy

Rigid bronchoscopes are long, straight hollow metal tubes that are inserted into the bronchus (see Fig. 5-14), usually for one of the following reasons:

- View airway abnormalities.
- Biopsy tissue or specimens for chronic infections or masses.
- Evaluate abnormal bleeding from the lungs.
- Remove foreign objects lodged in the airway.
- Open the spaces of a blocked airway.
- Treat bronchial stenosis (narrowing) with laser.
- Directly apply medication.

The set up for rigid bronchoscopy is similar to that of rigid laryngoscopy except that the scopes are longer. You need light cord or fibers, a light source box and suction. If tissue or specimens are anticipated, biopsy forceps, graspers or cup forceps should be available. A mouth guard should be placed over the patient's upper teeth prior to insertion of the scope to protect the teeth from damage.

Patient positioning varies according to institution or surgeon preference, but generally the patient is placed supine with a shoulder roll or doughnut headrest.

Rigid Esophagoscopy

Rigid esophagoscopy is used for direct visualization of the esophagus and top of the stomach. Like the rigid bronchoscopes, the rigid esophagoscopes are long, hollow, metal tubes that are inserted into the esophagus, usually for one of the following reasons:

- Visualize masses or lesions.

FIGURE 5–13 Rigid laryngoscope.

FIGURE 5–14 Rigid bronchoscopes.

- Remove foreign body; this is the most common reason this procedure is done in pediatrics.
- Inject esophageal varices.
- Obtain tissue or specimens for biopsy or examination.
- Dilate strictures or stenosis (narrowing).

The set up for rigid esophagoscopy is similar to that of rigid bronchoscopy except that the scopes are longer (see Fig. 5-15). You need light cord or fibers, a light source box and suction. If tissue or specimens are anticipated, biopsy forceps, graspers or cup forceps should be available. A mouth guard should be placed over the patient's upper teeth prior to insertion of the scope to protect the teeth from damage.

Patient positioning varies according to institution or surgeon preference, but generally the patient is placed supine with a shoulder roll or doughnut headrest.

Mediastinoscopy

The mediastinoscope is a lighted hollow metal tube with a handle attached at a right angle (see Fig. 5-16) used to look inside the space under the sternum between the lungs (the mediastinum). Located in this space are the large vessels, heart, lymph nodes, trachea and esophagus. A mediastinoscopy is usually done for one of the following reasons:

- Detect lymphoma (including Hodgkin's disease).
- Diagnose sarcoidosis.
- Biopsy masses or tumors.
- Stage cancer (including obtaining lymph nodes).
- Diagnose chronic infections.

As with other rigid endoscopes, a light source box is required and a camera may be attached to allow for viewing of the surgical field on a video monitor. Newer scopes have the camera built into the handle, which is less awkward and has a better picture quality than a separate attachment.

The patient is placed in a supine position with the head and neck hyperextended. An incision is made into the suprasternal notch for insertion of the scope.

Note: The making of an incision requires that the mediastinoscopy be treated as a sterile procedure rather than a

FIGURE 5-15 Rigid esophagoscopes.

FIGURE 5-16 Mediastinoscopy set. (Courtesy of http://www.entscope.com/servlet/the-template/about/Page).

surgically clean procedure like other endoscopes. Strict aseptic technique must be followed when handling supplies and instruments as well as when prepping and draping for this procedure. Failure to do so could result in postoperative infection and possible death of the patient.

Thoracoscope

The procedure abbreviated VATS (video-assisted thoracoscopic surgery) utilizes a rigid telescope and three to four ports to perform minimally invasive surgery on the lung (see Fig. 5-17). Two 10-mm scopes should be available: a 0 degree and a 30 degree. As with other endoscopic procedures, a light source box, camera and video monitor are required.

VATS is usually performed for one of the following reasons:

- Biopsy lung, pleura or diaphragm.
- Resect the lung.
- Decorticate the lung.
- Diagnose cancer or infection.
- Perform wedge resection of the lung.
- Perform pleurodesis for treatment of pneumothorax or pleural effusion.
- Perform sympathectomy or sympathotomy for treatment of hyperhidrosis (excessive sweating).

The patient is placed in a lateral position with the operative side upward. Follow all precautions for lateral positioning including proper padding of legs, ankles and arms; placement

FIGURE 5-17 Thoracoscopy set.

of an axillary roll and secure fastening of the patient to the bed.

Incisions are used to insert the ports for the camera and instruments; therefore, strict aseptic technique must be followed when handling supplies and instruments as well as prepping and draping for this procedure. Failure to do so could result in postoperative infection and possible death of the patient.

ARTHROSCOPY EQUIPMENT

The term *arthroscopy* means to look within a joint. Arthroscopes can be used to perform procedures of the shoulder, knee, hip, elbow, wrist and ankle (see Fig. 5-18). It has become one of the most common orthopedic procedures performed.

Arthroscopies are performed to diagnose and repair injury to a joint. Some of the most common arthroscopic procedures include ligament, tendon and cartilage repair; ligament replacement; foreign body removal; chondroplasty; rotator cuff surgery; impingement syndrome treatment and searching for the cause of chronic pain and swelling.

Equipment set up is much the same as for any other endoscopic procedure. You need an arthroscope, trocars or cannulas

(including an inflow cannula to instill fluid into the joint), one or two video monitors, a light source, arthroscopy pump and tubing, large (3000 cc) bags of normal saline for irrigation, large capacity suction device (e.g., Neptune or jug suction), camera, printer with paper, and electrocautery, hooks, probes, shavers, graspers and other instruments (depending on the procedure). *All* equipment and instruments must be checked before the start of the procedure to ensure that they are working. Make sure to check the printer for an adequate supply of paper.

Arthroscopic surgery requires a large amount of irrigation fluid. The fluid is pumped into the joint using an arthroscopy pump (see Fig. 5-4). There are many models of arthroscopy pumps available; make sure you are familiar with the pump(s) your institution uses. The pump should be set up and tested prior to the start of the procedure. If the pump is not pumping fluid properly, check the tubing to make sure it is inserted correctly and does not have a kink in it. If the pump still fails to pump properly, get another pump.

It is the responsibility of the circulator to keep an eye on the fluid level in the irrigation bag. Fluid should never be allowed to run out. Newer pumps have an alarm that signals a low fluid level, but do not rely solely on the alarm. Keep an eye on the fluid level and change the bag before it runs out.

It is the responsibility of the scrub person to check the arthroscope (see Fig. 5-19) and camera to make sure the picture is clear and that the lens or fibers are not broken or cracked. The scope should be checked to make sure it is not bent or damaged. All cords must be checked to make sure the fibers are not broken or that the casing is not cracked or damaged. Instruments should be checked to make sure they are in good working order (not difficult to open or close, not sticking).

Patient positioning depends on the procedure being performed. Knee arthroscopy usually requires the patient to be in a supine position with the affected knee in a holder that keeps it bent (e.g., knee-crutch stirrup), although some surgeons do not use the holder and just bend the knee with the foot flat on the bed. Depending on the procedure and the surgeon, shoulder arthroscopy can be performed with the patient supine with the affected arm suspended in traction or with the patient positioned sitting using a "beach chair" positioner. Hip arthroscopy can be performed with the patient positioned on a fracture bed, with the affected leg in traction. Make sure you have all the required positioning equipment available prior to bringing the patient into the OR room.

FIGURE 5-18 Shaver and arthroscopic instruments.

FIGURE 5-19 Arthroscope.

FLEXIBLE ENDOSCOPES

Flexible endoscopes are available for use in a variety of nonsurgical procedures. Bronchoscopy, esophagoscopy, endoscopic retrograde cholangiopancreaticography, gastroscopy, colonoscopy and sigmoidoscopy are the most common, but flexible endoscopes are available to perform hysteroscopy, cystoscopy, and rhinolaryngoscopy as well.

As its name implies, the flexible endoscope is a long, hollow, flexible tube with a light on the end (a light source box is required) and a camera attached that is used to inspect passageways within the body (see Fig. 5-20). Located within the scope are channels where biopsy, suction and irrigation instruments can be passed. The tip of the scope can be rotated 360 degrees to allow for complete visualization of tissue. The diameter and length of the tube varies depending on the intended use and on the size of the patient (pediatric or adult).

Flexible endoscopies are most commonly used to diagnose or treat problems within the digestive tract including the following:

- Abdominal pain
- Gastric ulcers
- Tumors, masses and polyps
- Intestinal tract bleeding (e.g., vomiting blood or passing blood rectally)
- Gastritis
- Common bile duct stones
- Changes in bowel habits
- Tissue retrieval for examination

The performance of flexible endoscopy alone does not (in most cases) require the use of anesthesia. Most procedures are performed with sedation and a topical anesthetic. As with any procedure, the scope, light source, video monitor and other equipment must be checked *prior* to the start of the procedure to make sure they are working properly.

Patient positioning depends on what procedure is being performed, with supine being the most common position for endoscopy of the upper tract and either side lying (Sims) or lithotomy for endoscopy of the lower tract.

FIGURE 5–20 Flexible scope.

Care of Flexible Endoscopes

As with any delicate (and expensive!) piece of equipment, care is needed when handling flexible endoscopes. Here are some general rules to follow when handling and cleaning flexible scopes, but be sure you read and are familiar with the manufacturer's instructions prior to using the scope:

- Flexible endoscopes contain fiberoptic bundles; coiling scopes too tightly can break the fibers.
- Do not place heavy instruments or equipment on top of the endoscope as it could damage the fiberoptic bundles or make a hole in the outer casing of the scope.
- Lay scopes on a flat surface when not in use to avoid kinking or twisting the shaft of the scope.
- Prior to use, inspect all scopes for holes or tears on the outer casing. Hook up all equipment to the scope and turn it on to make sure you have a clear picture (dark spots within the picture can be indicative of broken fiberoptic bundles).
- Prior to use, inspect all scopes to make sure they are free of bioburden.
- Clean bioburden (e.g., blood, secretions and feces) from the scope and instruments as needed during the procedure to ensure adequate visualization of the cavity. Wipe the scope immediately after use to prevent bioburden from drying on the scope.
- Follow the manufacturer's instructions for cleaning the scope. Soak the scope only if it is immersible. Clean all channels within the scope as well as all valves and ports. Long, thin soft brushes are available for cleaning hard to reach areas. Flush all channels, ports and valves clean after using the brush to loosen debris.
- Test all flexible scopes for leaks according to manufacturer's instructions.
- Rinse the scope with copious amounts of fresh water to remove debris and cleaning solution.
- Dry the scope according to manufacturer's instructions. All channels, ports and valves must be free of moisture.
- Routinely inspect all scopes for broken fiberoptic bundles, broken control switches or deflectors and leaks. Inspect lenses for scratches and looseness.
- Lay scopes flat or hang them up with the control handle in the upright position and the tube hanging downward for storage. They should not be stored near the edge of a table or where they could easily be bumped and damaged against something hard.

NEEDLES, TROCARS AND INSTRUMENTS

When a procedure of the abdomen or pelvis is going to be performed laparoscopically, the abdominopelvic cavity must first be filled with carbon dioxide, creating a *pneumoperitoneum*.

The purpose of the pneumoperitoneum is to help prevent injury to tissue and organs as well as to provide space for the insertion of trocars and instruments.

Carbon dioxide is used to inflate the abdomen because it readily available, is odorless, does not support combustion, has a lower incidence of embolism than air and is reabsorbed by the body.

To introduce carbon dioxide into the abdomen, the surgeon will use a *Veress needle* (also known as a *pneumoperitoneum needle*). Veress needles come in various lengths to accommodate patients of differing abdominal girths (see Fig. 5-21).

The usual technique for insertion of the Veress needle is for the surgeon to make a small "stab" incision into the upper abdominal tissues; lift up the skin with a Kocher, Backhaus or other penetrating clamp; and push the distal end of the needle through the tissue at an angle to avoid injuring underlying structures. The proximal end of needle is attached to insufflator tubing, which is attached to the insufflating control box (see Fig. 5-22). The tubing must have a filter and should be flushed with carbon dioxide (to remove air) prior to insufflation of the abdomen.

An alternative to using the Veress needle is for the surgeon to insert a *Hasson cannula* (see Fig. 5-23). This technique requires the surgeon to make a 1-cm incision in the area of the umbilicus and place a heavy suture into the fascia on each side of the incision. The surgeon then bluntly dissects down to the peritoneum, lifts the peritoneum with clamps and incises it.

The Hasson cannula (with a blunt obturator) is inserted into the abdominal cavity, taking care to protect the viscera. The sutures are wrapped around the locking tabs on the cannula to hold it in place. The insufflator tubing is attached to port on the cannula.

Once the abdomen is inflated, the surgeon makes several more small incisions that allow for the introduction of the trocar/cannula system (see Fig. 5-24). The trocar is the part of the device that pierces the tissue, whereas the cannula is the part that is left after the trocar is removed. The tip of the trocar can be blunt or sharp, although blunt trocars are now more common because they pose less threat of injury to internal organs. The cannula is used to create a port for introducing the camera or instruments into the internal cavity. The cannulas vary in size from 5 mm to 15 mm; 5 mm and 10 mm are the most commonly used sizes.

There are times when you may have a 10-mm trocar inserted into the abdomen, but the instrument you want to use is 5 mm. In that case, you place a *reducer* onto the trocar (see Fig. 5-25). This reducer has a soft, pliable opening that closes around the 5-mm instrument so that you do not lose carbon dioxide out of the abdomen. If you were just to insert a 5-mm instrument into a 10-mm trocar, there would be open space

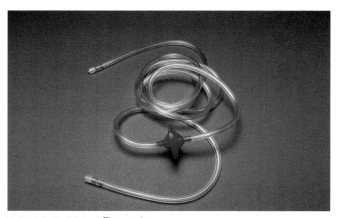
FIGURE 5-22 Insufflator tubing.

WATCH OUT! **Hypercarbia**

■ *Hypercarbia* is defined as excess carbon dioxide in the body.

■ Excess carbon dioxide in the body can create metabolic acidosis, leading to cardiac and respiratory abnormalities.

■ Despite the potential for hypercarbia, carbon dioxide remains the safest and most commonly used gas to create a pneumoperitoneum.

FIGURE 5-21 Veress needles.

FIGURE 5-23 Hasson cannula.

FIGURE 5-24 Trocar/cannula systems.

FIGURE 5-26 Laparoscopic instrument.

FIGURE 5-25 Reducer cap.

FIGURE 5-27 Laparoscopic instrument with cautery.

around the instrument that would allow the carbon dioxide to escape and decrease your pneumoperitoneum.

Instruments

If you look at the tips of laparoscopic instruments, they look very much like the tips of your common surgical instruments: allis, Kocher, hemostat, scissors, mixters, and so on. The difference lies in the shaft length and handle. Laparoscopic instruments have a long, narrow shaft and a trigger style handle (see Fig. 5-26). The long narrow shaft allows the instrument to be inserted through the cannula into the abdomen. The trigger style handle allows for more precise manipulation of the instrument. These instruments tend to be very delicate and should be handled with extra care. The length of the shaft makes it more susceptible to bending or breaking, the handle mechanisms can become too stiff or too loose to manipulate precisely and the tips can become loose, fall off or become damaged.

Laparoscopic instruments can be disposable or reusable. Some laparoscopic instruments have a place to attach an electrosurgery unit cord, allowing the instrument to be used for cauterization (see Fig. 5-27).

There are instruments that have a device near the handle that allows for rotation of the tip, making it so that the user can manipulate the tip without having to rotate the entire instrument (see Fig. 5-28).

Suturing inside the cavity during laparoscopic surgery always presents a challenge. There are several devices that are

FIGURE 5-28 Laparoscopic instrument with rotation device.

used for suturing and more being developed as this is being written. Each device has its own merits and drawbacks. The device used is generally based on what the surgeon is comfortable with and what tissue he or she is suturing.

Stapling devices are available for laparoscopic use. Just like standard instruments, there are laparoscopic stapling devices available that place a single staple (Ligaclip) or a row of staples (see Fig. 5-29). The tip of the stapler looks like the tip of a regular clip applier or stapler, but it is attached to a long, narrow shaft.

Laparoscopic irrigation devices consist of a long, thin tube that has multiple holes along the sides of the tip and at the end (see Fig. 5-30). Some of these devices are a combination of irrigation and suction with a hand control at the proximal end to allow the operator to switch between the two modes. Generally, 3000-cc bags of normal saline are attached to the device to use as an irrigating solution.

Suction devices need a power source: nitrogen or batteries. If using nitrogen, be sure to follow the manufacturer's recommendations for pressure setting; too low a pressure and the device will not work properly, too high a setting and it can cause the spike to come out of the bag and the whole bag of irrigation fluid will drain onto the floor!

FIGURE 5-30 A) and B) Laparoscopic irrigation devices.

FIGURE 5-29 Laparoscopic stapling devices. A) A single clip applier. B) A multiple staple applier.

Surgical Session Review

1) *Rhinoscopy* refers to viewing inside the:
   a. mouth
   b. nose
   c. ear
   d. throat

2) *Fluoroscopy* uses _____ to view inside tissues or organs.
   a. ultrasound waves
   b. laser
   c. x-ray
   d. electrical current

3) *Gastroscopy* refers to viewing inside the:
   a. small intestine
   b. large intestine
   c. esophagus
   d. stomach

4) Which of the following is *false* concerning a ureteroscope?
   a. The shaft is longer and thinner than a cystoscope.
   b. It can be rigid, semi-rigid or flexible.
   c. The shaft is shorter and thinner than a cystoscope.
   d. It is used to view inside the ureter.

5) The most common gas used to create a pneumoperitoneum is:
   a. carbon dioxide
   b. carbon monoxide
   c. oxygen
   d. helium

6) The gas pressure in the abdomen during laparoscopy should generally be around:
   a. 5 mm Hg
   b. 10 mm Hg
   c. 15 mm Hg
   d. 25 mm Hg

7) Video towers are not sterile; therefore, you need to make sure they are positioned at least _____ inches from the sterile drapes.
   a. 6-10
   b. 12-18
   c. 28-26
   d. 32-40

8) If the monitor video screen is dark, what should you check first?
   a. the fuses
   b. the power box to make sure it is not overloaded
   c. make sure it is plugged in and turned on
   d. make sure it is connected to the printer

9) Your patient is scheduled for a laryngoscopy. The surgeon will be looking inside the patient's _____.
   a. nose
   b. throat
   c. ear
   d. stomach

10) A mediastinoscopy can be used to aid in diagnosing:
    a. cervical cancer
    b. Hodgkin's disease
    c. AIDS
    d. Paget's disease

11) All of the following structures are located in the mediastinum *except* the:
    a. trachea
    b. heart
    c. esophagus
    d. lungs

12) Thoracoscopy can be performed for all of the following reasons *except:*
    a. lung biopsy
    b. wedge resection of the long
    c. decortication
    d. pneumonectomy

13) The acronym VATS means:
    a. Video- activated thoracoscopic surgery
    b. Video- assisted thoracoscopic surgery
    c. Video- aided thoracic surgery
    d. Video- aligned thoracic surgery

14) To avoid possible damage, cystoscopes should be handled by the:
    a. middle of the shaft
    b. tip end of the shaft
    c. light cable connector
    d. bridge

15) The patient is undergoing a TURBT that will involve electrocautery of bladder tumors. Which irrigation fluid would you anticipate using?
    a. normal saline
    b. dextrose in water
    c. lactated Ringer's
    d. glycine

16) _____ is the most common position for a patient undergoing cystoscopy.
a. supine
b. prone
c. Kraske
d. lithotomy

17) Arthroscopy can be used for all of the following *except:*
a. ligament damage repair
b. tendon damage repair
c. bone fractures
d. chondroplasty

18) The needle used to insert gas into the abdomen is known as a _____ needle.
a. Veress
b. Vegan
c. Vargan
d. Verrin

19) Excess carbon dioxide in the body is known as:
a. hypoxia
b. hypocarbia
c. hypercarbia
d. hyperglycemia

20) The three most common types of cystoscopes used have _____ degree tips.
a. 0, 30, 70
b. 0, 30, 65
c. 0. 20, 70
d. 10, 30, 70

CHAPTER 6

Lasers

Lasers are a relatively new technology in the surgical field, first used in the 1960s. Like all technology, lasers have vastly improved since their inception, allowing them to play a major role many surgical specialties.

The acronym *LASER* stands for light amplification by stimulated emission of radiation. Lasers work with light waves. Waves of light stimulate atoms to produce more waves of light until millions of waves of light produce an intense beam. This intense beam is used to vaporize or cut tissue or to control bleeding.

There are several factors that determine how deeply the beam penetrates into the tissue. These factors are power, color, wavelength, duration of tissue exposure and tissue consistency.

When laser light hits a surface (e.g., tissue) any of the following things can occur:

- *Reflection:* The direction of the beam is changed after it contacts a surface; the beam can be intentionally reflected to treat hard to reach areas or reflection can inadvertently happen and pose a safety hazard.
- *Scattering:* The beam can disperse in all directions, causing a decrease in intensity; the beam spreads over a large area.
- *Absorption:* The beam alters or disrupts the tissue in some way.
- *Transmission:* The beam is transmitted through tissue without thermally affecting it.

In order to produce these light waves, the laser needs an energy source or medium. It is this medium that gives each type of laser beam its distinct properties. Media can include gas, solid, liquid or semiconductor. The two media most commonly found in surgery are gas (i.e., argon, carbon dioxide and krypton) and solid (i.e., holmium, neodymium: yttrium–aluminum–garnet [Nd:YAG], potassium–titanyl–phosphate [KTP], dye and ruby). The laser is named after the medium that it contains.

Characteristics of LASER Beams

Even though they are produced by different mediums (e.g., gas, solid, dye excimer), all laser beams have certain common characteristics:

- *Coherent:* The peaks and troughs of the light wave are all exactly the same; the waves all travel in the same direction.
- *Monochromatic:* The light waves have all the same wavelength or color.
- *Parallel (collimated):* The light waves all move in narrow columns and do not spread out as they travel.

TYPES OF LASERS

The laser the surgeon chooses depends on the tissue on which it is to be used and the desired effect on that tissue. The next several paragraphs cover the most common types of lasers used in surgery, their effect on tissues and some of the types of surgery for which each is used.

Carbon Dioxide Laser

The *carbon dioxide* laser is the medical laser most commonly used in surgery (see Fig. 6-1). The beam from this laser is strongly absorbed by water, which constitutes a large portion of soft tissue, making the carbon dioxide laser suitable for a wide variety of surgeries. The absorption does not depend on tissue pigment; therefore, it can be used on light or dark tissue. The beam can be focused into a thin beam to cut tissue, similar to a conventional scalpel, or defocused to vaporize, ablate or shave tissue. This type of laser also can be used to coagulate bleeding vessels.

FIGURE 6-1 Carbon dioxide laser.

FIGURE 6-2 Argon laser.

FIGURE 6-3 Holmium laser.

Unlike other lasers, the *action* on the tissue is directly visible as it is being used. The beam itself, however, is invisible and requires a helium-neon beam (which is red) to make it visible for aiming purposes. The carbon dioxide laser has a wide variety of uses in many surgical specialties including laparoscopic gynecological surgeries, wart ablation, laryngectomy, benign laryngeal lesions, middle ear procedures, skin lesion removal, breast biopsy, breast reduction, tumor removal from the brain and spinal cord, skin resurfacing (for irregularities or wrinkles), vascular surgeries and some podiatry surgeries.

Argon Laser

The *argon* laser produces a visible blue-green beam that is absorbed by red-brown pigmented tissues (e.g., hemoglobin and melanin) (see Fig. 6-2). This type of beam is not absorbed by clear tissue, making it useful for retinal surgery because it passes through the cornea, vitreous and lens of the eye without any effect on them.

Argon lasers are used for sealing and coagulation. Uses for argon lasers include treatment of port wine stains, dark moles or lesions, spider veins on the face, retinopathy, glaucoma and inner ear surgery.

Holmium:YAG Laser

A third type of laser used in surgery is the *holmium:YAG* (also referred to as a *holmium* laser) (see Fig. 6-3). The acronym YAG stands for *yttrium-aluminum-garnet*, which is used in combination with other mediums in laser therapy.

The holmium laser has a beam outside of the visible range; therefore, an aiming beam is necessary to see where the laser will hit the tissue. The aiming beam may be red or green.

The holmium laser is versatile as it can cut, ablate, coagulate and contour tissues of all types. It can be used in urology to perform laser lithotripsy on renal stones or to resect prostate tissue, in orthopedics to ablate bone or cartilage, in ear nose throat (ENT) surgery to assist with endoscopic sinus procedures or in endoscopic spinal surgery to remove a disk. In addition to these applications, it can be used in gynecological surgery, general surgery and ophthalmology (to perform laser thermal keratoplasty to treat farsightedness).

Neodymium:YAG Laser

Neodymium is another medium that is used in conjunction with yttrium-aluminum-garnet and is referred to as an *Nd:YAG* laser. Like the holmium:YAG laser, the Nd:YAG laser has a beam that is outside the visible range and needs an aiming beam (usually a red helium-neon beam).

This type of laser is absorbed by pigmented tissues and has the greatest ability of any laser to coagulate blood vessels. The Nd:YAG laser can be used in ophthalmology to perform iridotomy or to treat diabetic retinopathy, in cosmetic surgery to remove hair or to treat spider veins, and in dental surgery to perform certain procedures on the soft tissues (e.g., gingivectomy). There are some dual wavelength Nd:YAG lasers available that can be used for general, orthopedic, ENT, thoracic and podiatry procedures.

OTHER TYPES OF LASERS

This section describes lasers that are less common to surgical procedures.

The *excimer* laser uses a combination of an inert gas (e.g., krypton, xenon or argon) and a reactive gas (e.g., chlorine or fluorine). It emits short bursts of laser light through fiberoptic cables that cause tissue to disintegrate (ablation). This type of laser creates less heat than others, thus making it less damaging to nearby tissues. It is extremely precise; able to remove 0.25 μm of tissue with a single pulse. The main uses for this laser are LASIK (laser-assisted in situ keratomileusis) eye surgery and photorefractive keratotomy.

The *ruby* laser was one of the first lasers used for medical procedures. The ruby medium is a solid crystal made from aluminum oxide and chromium atoms that are activated by flash-lamps in the resonator cavity to produce the beam. This beam is strongly absorbed by blue and black pigment and melanin but not by transparent substances or oxyhemoglobin. The ruby laser is used to remove port wine stains, freckles, liver spots and dark nevi as well as tattoos.

The *KTP* (potassium-titanyl-phosphate) laser produces a green light that is used to cut tissue, treat vascular lesions (leg veins) and remove red and orange tattoo pigment. It is also used to treat rosacea and port wine stains and, recently, has been used to vaporize prostate tissue.

Tunable dye lasers emit a pulsed laser beam that is produced when certain dyes or vapors are exposed to argon laser light. The dye absorbs the light and produces a broad-spectrum light that is tuned to produce a beam of a particular color (wavelength). This type of laser is used to destroy vascular (e.g., port wine stains, rosacea, cherry angiomas) and pigmented (e.g., café-au-lait spots, nevi) lesions. Another use of tunable dye lasers is photosensitive drug therapy (PDT). In PDT, a photosensitive dye is injected about 48 hours prior to surgery, the dye is metabolized out of normal tissue but remains in malignant tissue and the laser is used to destroy the malignant tissue.

As laser technology improves, the medical and surgical applications for it broaden. Some of the advantages to laser procedures include shorter hospital stays, less painful recoveries and less blood in the surgical field (meaning better visualization).

Although they do have advantages, medical lasers are powerful machines capable of doing great harm to patients and personnel if used improperly. The next section covers the general important safety rules to follow when using lasers.

LASER SAFETY

Due to the intense nature of laser beams, if they are not used properly they have the potential to cause great harm: fire, electrical shock, and damage to unintended tissues (or persons!).

The use of laser technology is regulated by several government agencies. The job of these agencies is to put into place regulations to ensure the safety of patients and staff while lasers are in use. The three agencies that develop and oversee

regulations for lasers used in medicine are the Occupational Safety and Health Administration (OSHA), the American National Standards Institute (ANSI) and the Center for Devices and Radiological Health (CDRH).

In addition to these agencies, each institution has policies and procedures to deal with the safe use of lasers within their own facility, including designating a laser safety officer in the operating room (OR) and credentialing those permitted to operate using lasers. The Association of periOperative Registered Nurses (AORN) has published guidelines for laser safety, which many institutions use as a basis for their own procedures for the safe use of lasers in the OR setting.

Although each institution has its own set of policies dealing with laser safety, there are some basic rules that should be followed to ensure safe use of lasers. Make sure you know your own institution's policies and procedures:

- All doorways leading into the room where a laser is in use must be marked with a warning sign stating that a laser is in use (see Fig. 6-4).
- Eye tissue is the most vulnerable of all tissues to inadvertent exposure. All personnel who enter into the room must wear proper protective eyewear. Each type of laser requires eyewear that protects against inadvertent eye exposure to that specific type of laser beam. Make sure that the eyewear in the room is specific to the type of laser being used (e.g., eyewear designed for use with a carbon dioxide laser will NOT protect your eyes against inadvertent exposure to a beam from a holmium laser).
- Proper eyewear needs to be posted on the outer door or just outside the room for use by those who enter the room for any reason.
- Patient's eyes need to be protected against inadvertent exposure. Patients should be fitted with the same eyewear that the staff is wearing (some institutions have protective eye cups that are used for this purpose).
- Regular eyeglasses or goggles are NOT protective eyewear. The eyewear must be specifically designed

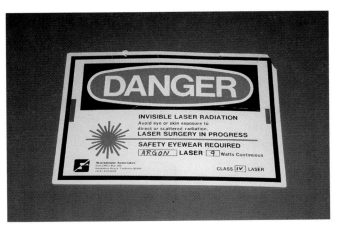

FIGURE 6-4 Laser safety door sign.

for the laser being used and cover the tops, bottoms and sides of the eye to offer complete protection (see Fig. 6-5).

■ Only personnel knowledgeable in the use and operation of lasers and in laser safety protocols should be allowed to operate the laser. Ongoing education should be in place for staff regarding the safe use of lasers.

■ Laser surgery should be performed only by those surgeons credentialed or approved by the institution to do so.

■ The foot pedal for turning the laser beam on and off should ONLY be operated by the surgeon holding the handpiece. The pedal should NOT be operated by an assistant, scrub or nurse.

■ All electrical cords should be inspected prior to surgery. If a cord is found to be frayed or otherwise compromised, the laser should NOT be used until it is inspected and repaired by the biomedical engineering department.

■ When not in use during surgery, the laser should be placed in "standby" mode.

■ There should be a designated laser nurse to operate the machine during the procedure. He or she should stand next to the machine to place it in "standby" mode when not in use and "ready" mode when the surgeon is ready to use it.

■ Fire safety precautions must be followed. These include:

　■ Allow all prep solutions to dry completely before using the laser.

　■ Surround the surgical site with wet towels.

　■ Use nonreflective instruments.

　■ Use special laser endotracheal tubes if the laser will be used anywhere near the airway.

　■ Use flame-retardant drapes.

　■ When not in use, the tip of the laser should be placed on a moist towel not a dry drape.

■ Oxygen should be delivered at the lowest possible concentration.

■ Water or saline must be available on the surgical field (usually on the back table).

■ Portable fire extinguishers must be readily available (halon extinguishers are recommended).

■ Nonexplosive anesthetics must be used.

■ During anorectal procedures, the rectum must be packed with a sterile water-soaked sponge to prevent a methane gas fire.

■ Liquids should NOT be placed on top of the laser machine (they could spill and cause a fire or electrical short).

■ All surfaces in the room must be nonreflective, all tables should be covered or removed from the room, all instruments should be nonreflective (matte finish or ebony), metal jewelry should not be worn by personnel in the room or entering the room.

■ A laser safety officer should be designated to update and enforce laser safety policies.

■ To protect against plume exposure, staff should wear specially designated laser masks (these masks are designed to filter smaller particles of matter).

■ Smoke evacuators (not just regular suction) should be used to suction and filter the plume that is produced. The filters in these units need to be checked and changed according to manufacturer's instructions.

■ When storing the laser, the key should NOT be left in the machine.

■ Shades should be pulled to cover room windows (or cover windows with nonreflective material) to prevent beam reflection or, in some cases, beam penetration through the glass to outside the room.

The use of lasers in surgery has become commonplace. It is up to *every* staff member to know what the safety protocols and policies are and to see that they are followed. The safety of your patient, your coworkers and yourself depends on it.

FIGURE 6–5 Laser eyewear.

Troubleshooting Tips

As with any device, troubleshooting starts with the seemingly obvious and simple (see Figs. 6-6 and 6-7):

- Make sure the machine is plugged in.
- Make sure the machine is turned on.
- Check to see that the machine is in "ready" mode, not "standby"

After checking that the items in this bulleted list are done, start to look for the problem.

PROBLEM	WHAT TO LOOK AT
No beam comes out of the fiber.	■ Is the fiber plugged into the machine? ■ Is the connection between the fiber and machine tight? ■ Is the machine on "ready" (not "standby")? ■ Is the foot pedal connected to the machine? ■ Does the fiber need to be replaced?
The beam is misaligned.	■ The beam should be checked according to institution policy before use to check for misalignment. If the beam is misaligned, the machine should be checked by qualified service personnel; the mirrors may have been damaged or moved during moving of the laser from one place to another.
The beam is not "crisp" (it has a star or scattered look to it).	■ If using a reusable fiber, the fiber may need to be recut and stripped; see manufacturer's instructions on how to do this.
The laser has low power.	■ Check all beam delivery optics. Make sure they are free of dust, dirt and smoke
The power does not come on.	■ Is the machine plugged in— you may need to try a different wall plug ■ Is the power switch in the "on" position? ■ Is the key in the ignition and the ignition turned to "on"? ■ Is the "dummy switch" located in the back of the laser missing?

FIGURE 6-6 Laser control panel.

FIGURE 6-7 A) Laser with the dummy switch in place. B) The dummy switch is missing.

Surgical Session Review

1) All of the following are characteristics of laser light *except:*
   a. monochromatic
   b. coherent
   c. polychromatic
   d. collimated

2) Which factor(s) effect how deep the laser beam penetrates?
   a. duration of tissue exposure
   b. power
   c. wavelength
   d. all of the above

3) Scattering of a laser beam as it hits a surface (e.g., tissue) can cause:
   a. an increase in intensity
   b. a narrowing of the beam
   c. a decrease in intensity
   d. the beam to spread over a smaller area

4) The changing of the direction of the laser as it contacts a surface is known as:
   a. scattering
   b. reflection
   c. absorption
   d. transmission

5) The energy source for the laser is known as a *medium.* All of the following can be forms of media *except:*
   a. gas
   b. solid
   c. semiconductor
   d. steam

6) An example of a solid laser medium is:
   a. argon
   b. holmium
   c. carbon dioxide
   d. krypton

7) The most commonly used medical laser is:
   a. carbon dioxide
   b. argon
   c. ruby
   d. holmium

8) Which of the following lasers *does not* require an aiming beam?
   a. carbon dioxide
   b. holmium
   c. argon
   d. Nd:YAG

9) Which of the following are potential hazards of laser use?
   a. fire
   b. electrical shock
   c. damage to unintended tissue
   d. all of the above

10) Which agency *regulates* the use of medical lasers in the workplace?
   a. AST
   b. AORN
   c. ANSI
   d. AMA

11) All of the following statements are true about laser protective eyewear *except:*
   a. Laser eyewear should be posted on the outside of the door of the room in case someone needs to enter the room.
   b. Each eyewear is specific for a certain type of beam; therefore, you must check to make sure you have the eyewear specific to the laser you are using.
   c. Patients do not need to have their eyes protected because they are behind the drape.
   d. Regular eyeglasses or goggles are not considered protective eyewear.

12) The laser foot pedal should *only* be operated by the:
   a. assistant
   b. scrub
   c. circulator
   d. surgeon holding the handpiece

13) During the procedure, when the laser in not in use, it should be placed in the _____ mode.
   a. standby
   b. ready
   c. coagulating
   d. cutting

14) Fire safety precautions for laser use include:
   a. using flame-retardant drapes
   b. using non-reflective instruments
   c. surrounding the surgical site with wet towels
   d. all of the above

15) All surfaces in the room must be:
   a. reflective
   b. nonreflective
   c. sterile
   d. nonsterile

16) Who is responsible for updating and enforcing laser safety policies?
   a. the surgeon
   b. the physician assistant
   c. the laser safety officer
   d. the hospital CEO

17) When storing the laser, the key should be:
   a. hidden
   b. stored in the machine
   c. not stored in the machine
   d. left in the ignition

18) The laser machine does not come on. You have checked; the machine is plugged in, the power switch is in the "on" position, the key is in the ignition and the ignition is in the "on" position. What could be the likely problem?
   a. a hospital-wide power outage
   b. the dummy switch in the back is missing
   c. the fiber is faulty
   d. the fiber needs to be recut

19) One of the main uses for an excimer laser is:
   a. gynecological surgery
   b. orthopedic surgery
   c. LASIK surgery
   d. neurosurgery

20) Which type of laser has a beam that is not absorbed by clear tissue, making it useful for retinal surgery?
   a. carbon dioxide
   b. argon
   c. holmium
   d. ruby

CHAPTER 7

Specialty Equipment

NEUROSURGERY EQUIPMENT

Neurosurgery, specifically surgery on the brain, requires specialized equipment, and it is essential for operating room (OR) personnel to be familiar with it. In Chapter 1, some of the specific positioning devices (e.g., Mayo headrest) and furniture (e.g., large Mayo stand and overhead table) are described. Chapters 2 and 3 include some specific supplies (e.g., neuro patties or cottonoids) and drains (e.g., ventricular drain). In this section, some of the equipment used for surgery on the brain is described.

Cranial Access Kit

The disposable cranial access kit (see Fig. 7-1) is used to perform emergency or bedside *ventriculostomy* (burr hole access into the cranium). A ventriculostomy is performed in order to monitor intracranial pressure (ICP) or to drain cerebrospinal fluid or blood from the central nervous system to relieve pressure.

This kit is designed for single patient use. Although contents of the kits vary, most of them include a hand drill and drill bits, prepping supplies (including razors and prep solution), drapes, scissors, suturing equipment, tubes for collecting cerebrospinal fluid samples, disposable scalpels, needles, syringes and local anesthetic.

Intracranial Pressure Monitor

The ICP monitor (see Fig. 7-2) is used to continuously monitor the pressure surrounding the brain. Patients requiring ICP monitoring include those who have sustained head trauma or brain hemorrhage, those who have undergone brain surgery and those who have cranial tumors.

A small plastic tube is inserted into the brain, usually in the top left or right portion. The tube is connected to a monitor that continuously displays ICP. Normal ICP in an adult is 8 to 18 mm Hg. An increased pressure reading could be indicative of brain swelling, which could lead to herniation or permanent neurological damage if uncorrected. Complications of ICP monitor insertion include infection or hemorrhage.

Cavitron Ultrasonic Surgical Aspirator/Sonopet

The Cavitron Ultrasonic Surgical Aspirator (CUSA) is a device designed to break up and remove specific types of brain tumors. The device uses ultrasonic waves to fragment the tumor and then removes it by irrigation and suction.

Similar to the CUSA is the Sonopet machine (see Fig. 7-3). The Sonopet also uses ultrasonic waves to fragment brain tumors and removes them through suction and irrigation. It is also a bone cutting aspirator. Unlike conventional cranial sawing devices, there is minimal heat generation at the tip when cutting bone.

There are many tips available for the handpieces of both devices to allow for use on a variety of tumor types and locations. The Sonopet machine also has a variety of bone cutting tips available.

Image Guidance System

The image guidance system (also known as the *stealth station system* or the *stealth*) is a system that takes computed tomography

FIGURE 7–1 Cranial access kit.

FIGURE 7–2 ICP monitor kit.

FIGURE 7–3 Sonopet machine.

FIGURE 7–4 Stealth station machine.

(CT) scan, ultrasound, magnetic resonance imaging (MRI) or conventional radiograph images and transforms them into three-dimensional (3-D) images (see Fig. 7-4). The 3-D images allow the surgeon to know the exact location of the lesion or tissue to be removed. These images can be rotated and manipulated to give the surgeon the exact view needed. These images can be taken prior to surgery to aid in pre-procedure planning or intraoperatively.

These systems have been developed for use in *neurosurgery* (removal of brain tumors and spinal procedures), ear nose throat (ENT) procedures (polypectomy, functional endoscopic sinus surgery [FESS], cholesteatomas) and orthopedic procedures (total knee or hip and trauma).

The image is projected on a touch screen monitor. The use of special instruments allows the surgeon to register the location of the instrument in relation to the location of the lesion. The image on the screen shows where the instrument is situated so that the surgeon can protect surrounding tissue and blood vessels. For example, during polyp surgery, the ENT surgeon can see, within 1 mm, where the instrument is in relation to the brain, thus allowing the surgeon to extract more polyp tissue without fear of inadvertently causing damage or contamination to the brain.

Like any technology, the use of machines requires that OR personnel know how to load images into the machine, set up and position the machine in the room, and troubleshoot the equipment during a procedure. Personnel must make sure that they are knowledgeable about manufacturer's instructions and

recommendations on equipment function prior to being assigned to a case.

CARDIOPULMONARY BYPASS MACHINE

The cardiopulmonary bypass machine, also known as the *heart-lung machine* or *pump oxygenator,* is used to replace the heart and lungs during some cardiac surgery procedures. The machine gathers the blood, removes excess carbon dioxide, oxygenates it and returns it to the body. In addition, the machine filters the blood and controls its temperature. Cardiopulmonary bypass is used during many cardiac procedures including the following:

- Coronary artery bypass graft (CABG)
- Heart or heart-lung transplant
- Heart valve replacement or repair
- Birth defect repair (e.g., septal defects, tetralogy of Fallot, transposition of great vessels)
- Pulmonary thrombolectomy
- Large aortic aneurysm repair
- Rewarming of severe hypothermia victims

The cardiopulmonary bypass machine is operated by a perfusionist. He or she is a specially educated, having 2 to 4 years of undergraduate training before enrolling in a 2-year perfusion training program. The perfusionist is responsible for supporting the metabolic and physiologic needs of the patient while he or she is on the bypass machine, for monitoring physiologic parameters (e.g., blood gases, acid base balance, electrolytes and anticoagulation), for adjusting machine parameters as needed and for collecting autologous blood. Perfusionists monitor the pump lines for the presence of air. Any air must be removed immediately to prevent possible air embolus or stroke. All lines must be monitored to make sure none becomes disconnected from the machine as a patient could quickly exsanguinate from a disconnected line.

Special cannulae (see Fig. 7-5) are inserted into the vena cava and the ascending aorta, and the pump tubing is attached to the cannulae. The blood is taken out of the body via the cannula in the vena cava (or right atrium), which is called the *venous cannula*. This cannula is straight-ended with multiple holes in the tip. The blood is returned to the body through the aortic cannula. The aortic cannula may have a straight or angled tip. The femoral artery and femoral vein occasionally are used to collect and return the blood, generally when the great vessels cannot be used. The femoral artery catheter is tapered and has a beveled end for ease of insertion.

Cardiopulmonary bypass can be total or partial. *Total cardiopulmonary bypass* means that all the blood returning to the heart is forced into the venous cannula and out to the heart-lung machine (see Fig. 7-6). Total cardiopulmonary bypass is used for many cardiac surgeries: CABG, transplants, repair of most cardiac birth defects and valve replacements.

Partial cardiopulmonary bypass means that some blood is allowed to flow into the heart and "normal" circulation while the rest of the blood is diverted into the machine. Partial cardiopulmonary bypass can be used during some types of cardiothoracic surgery (e.g., repairs of some aortic anomalies) and as a temporary measure after coronary bypass grafting to wean the patient from the bypass machine.

BONE SCREWS, PLATES, NAILS, RODS, PINS AND STAPLES

Screws, plates, nails, rods and pins are used in orthopedic surgery to repair and stabilize fractures. Staples are used to reconnect soft

FIGURE 7-6 Heart-lung machine.

tissue to bone. This section covers the care and use of these devices.

All of these devices are considered implants because they are inserted into the bone or tissue and left inside the patient. Most of the time these implants are permanent, although some can removed after the fracture heals if they are bothersome to the patient (e.g., causing pain or discomfort).

Staples

The primary use of fixation staples is to reconnect soft tissue to bone, including anterior cruciate ligament repair. Other uses include tendon and ligament repair, bone fragment fixation and bone growth control.

Staples come in a variety of sizes and types (two, three or four prongs) to accommodate surgery on all types and sizes of bone and tissue (see Fig. 7-7). Most staples are straight, but some have an offset to allow for stable fixation of an osteotomy that has steps. There are staples available for use during open or arthroscopic procedures.

Staples are commonly made of stainless steel, but some are made from chromium-cobalt and nitinol alloy.

Staples are inserted with a staple driver and a mallet.

Nails and Rods

Nails and rods are used to fix fractures of long bones (i.e., femur, tibia and humerus) (see Fig. 7-8). They are driven into the

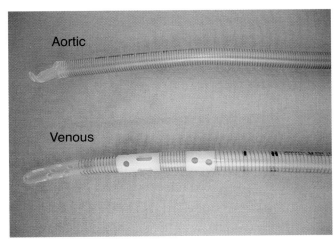

FIGURE 7-5 Cardiopulmonary cannulae.

WATCH OUT! Handling of Implants

- Any implant used must be documented in the patient's intraoperative record.

- Implants should be handled as little as possible to avoid possible contamination.

- If an implant must be flash sterilized (not recommended but sometimes necessary), a biological indicator must be flashed along with the implant. A chemical paper indicator is *not* sufficient.

- The circulator should double check the implant size and type with the surgeon before opening the package. Implants are very expensive; you must make sure you have the correct one before opening it onto the sterile field.

- Scrub personnel should always *measure* any screws prior to handing them to the surgeon. Do not rely on the numbers on the package or on the side of the tray. Mistakes happen and a screw could end up in the wrong section of the tray.

- Scrub personnel should double check pin size prior to handing pins to the surgeon. Trays could have been restocked incorrectly.

- Never reuse an implant. They are single-use devices. Reuse could weaken them.

- Do not use any implant that has been damaged; get a new one. Implants that are dropped, scratched or dented need to be discarded.

- Bending plates to conform to the bone should be avoided whenever possible. If a plate must be bent, a proper plate bending instrument should be used, not a pair of pliers.

- Implants of the same metal or alloy should be for the surgery. If implants of differing alloys are used, they can corrode and cause implant breakdown.

medullary canal to span the fracture sites. There are several manufacturers of these devices; make sure you are familiar with both the implant and the insertion instrument system being used by your institution.

Tibial nails are used to fix fractures of the large bone of the lower leg. The nails are designed to be used reamed or unreamed. Locking screws are inserted to hold them in place. They vary in diameter from 8 mm to 14 mm and are available

FIGURE 7-7 Fixation staples.

FIGURE 7-8 Nails.

in 26-cm through 42-cm lengths. They are made of stainless steel or a titanium alloy.

Humeral nails are used to repair fractures of the long bone of the upper arm. Most are designed to be inserted at either the elbow or the shoulder. There are two main styles of humeral nails: one style has a bend at the proximal end and is used to repair fractures of the proximal third of the humerus, whereas the other style is straight and is used to repair fractures of the shaft of the humerus. Some humeral nails have a flexible head and could be used to repair fractures anywhere in the humerus. The nails are held in place with a locking screw system. Humeral nails are available in 6-mm to 13-mm diameters and 18-cm to 30-cm lengths.

The intramedullary (IM) rod or nail is used to repair and align fractures of the femur. The rod is inserted into the bone marrow canal (IM canal). This allows the rod to share the weight-bearing load with the bone, making it possible for the patient to be mobile sooner. Femoral nails are available as antegrade, retrograde, Uniflex or distal, depending on the type of fracture they are being used to repair. Most femoral nails are available in 10-mm to 16-mm diameters and lengths ranging from 16 cm to 44 cm. Distal femoral nails are available in 9-mm to 13-mm diameters and 160-mm to 460-mm lengths. Rods and nails are generally made of titanium or a titanium alloy.

Bone Plates

Plates, along with screws, are used to traverse the surfaces of two bone fragments. Plates and screws can be used to repair fractures or stabilize bones (e.g., spinal surgery). Plates come in a variety of sizes and shapes to accommodate a variety of bone surfaces and sizes (see Fig. 7-9). Plates are used in cranial surgery (e.g., holding craniotomy bone flap in place), maxillofacial surgery (e.g., repair fractures of the jaw, facial bones and zygoma), orthopedic surgery (e.g., repair of fractures) and spinal surgery (e.g., stabilization of vertebrae). Plates generally are made of titanium, titanium/nickel alloy

FIGURE 7–9 Bone plates.

or stainless steel. As a general rule, it is best to avoid bending plates because this can weaken the metal, but if a plate must be bent to fit the fracture site, a plate bender made specifically for that purpose must be used. Plates come with anywhere from 2 to 12 holes, depending on the length, and in a variety of shapes.

Bone Screws

Bone screws can be used to attach a plate or soft tissue to bone, or they can be placed directly across the fracture ends of small bone fractures to repair them. There are two types of bone screw: *cancellous* and *cortical* (see Fig. 7-10). The screws' names are based on the type of bone on which they are designed to be used. It is very important that OR personnel be able to differentiate between the two types of screws so that the correct screw is available to the surgeon.

The cancellous screw has threads about two thirds of the way up the screw (this area is called the *shank*), then a non-threaded area of shaft. Cortical screws have threads all the way up the shank to the head of the screw.

Screws can be self-tapping or they may require that you use a "tap" (non–self-tapping) to make ridges in the bone for

the screw to follow. There are four steps for screw insertion with which scrub personnel should be familiar in order to anticipate what will be needed next:

1. *Drill:* Make a hole with a drill bit that is a smaller diameter than the screw being used.
2. *Measure:* Use a depth gauge to determine the length of the screw needed
3. *Tap:* Use a bone tap to create ridges for the screw to follow (not necessary if self-tapping screws are used).
4. *Screw:* Set the screw in place using a screwdriver.

To remember the steps for screw insertion I once heard someone use the pneumonic "**D**on't **M**arry **T**oo **S**oon" to stand for *drill, measure, tap, screw.*

Screws are commonly made from titanium, stainless steel or cobalt-chromium alloy. Cortical screws are available in 1.5-mm to 5.0-mm diameters and 6-mm to 110-mm lengths. Cancellous screws are available in 3.5-mm to 6.5-mm diameters and 10-mm to 110-mm lengths (thread length, 5 mm to 32 mm).

VITRECTOMY/CATARACT REMOVAL MACHINES

A vitrectomy is an ophthalmic operation that can be performed to remove scar tissue, repair retinal damage or detachment, clear blood and debris from the eye, repair a macular hole, or repair injury to the eye resulting from previous surgery.

During surgery for retinal detachment, the surgeon uses either *diathermy* (heat) or *cryothermy* (cold) to create adhesions (scar tissue) between the layers of tissue and repair the detachment. The detached area adheres to the scar tissue as it heals with the goal being for the damaged tissue to return to its normal position. A scleral buckle (small silicone or foam band) is attached to the sclera, causing it to indent and come in close contact with the retina during healing. The vitreous of the eye may be removed and replaced with a gas bubble or silicone oil. The oil or gas holds the retina in place and prevents traction or pulling on the newly repaired retina.

There are a few pieces of important machinery with which OR personnel must be familiar: the vitrectomy machine, the cryotherapy machine, the phacoemulsifier, and the laser (see Chapter 6 for information about lasers).

Vitrectomy Machine

Many of the newer vitrectomy machines (see Fig. 7-11) are capable of allowing the surgeon to perform procedures in the anterior or posterior chamber as well as to perform "combined" procedures involving cataract excision and vitreoretinal surgery. The machines are capable of phacoemulsification, diathermy and vitreous removal. They offer cutting, irrigation, aspiration, vacuum and viscous fluid control mode options.

Any vitrectomy machine requires set up time. It is the responsibility of the OR personnel assigned to the room to be

FIGURE 7–10 Cancellous and cortical bone screws.

FIGURE 7-11 A) Vitrectomy machine. B) Probe.

familiar with the machine, probes, tubing and irrigation set up for the machine used at their institution. Make sure to be familiar with manufacturer's guidelines for priming of tubing and probe or instrument attachment as well as the various modes at which the machine can be set.

Cryotherapy Machine

Cryotherapy is the use of extreme cold to freeze tissue. This therapy is used to treat retinal detachment by freezing the scleral tissue at the area(s) where the retina is detached without damage to adjacent tissue. It can also be used for some forms of cataract extraction.

An insulated probe is attached to the machine (see Fig. 7-12) and the cold is delivered to the tissue. The type of probe used

FIGURE 7-12 Cryotherapy machine.

depends on the surgical procedure. Probes are available for the following:

- Retinal surgery (treatment of detachment)
- Cataract surgery
- Trichiasis (ingrown eyelashes) treatment
- Endocryocoagulation
- Dislocated lens removal or repositioning
- Intravitreal foreign body removal

Phacoemulsifier

The phacoemulsifier (also referred to as the *phaco*) is used during cataract extraction (see Fig. 7-13). This machine uses ultrasonic energy, at a speed of about 40,000 cycles per second, to fragment the affected lens into tiny pieces while irrigating and suctioning to remove the pieces. This allows the lens to be removed using a very tiny incision, which in most cases does not require suturing. The tiny incision causes less trauma to the eye than open surgery and allows the procedure to be performed in about 15 minutes.

OR personnel are responsible for setting up and running the phacoemulsifier. There are several models of machines available; make sure you are familiar with the machine available in your institution prior to the procedure. All phacoemulsifiers require the use of irrigating solution, usually balanced saline solution (BSS). In addition to irrigating lens fragments, the BSS helps to maintain intraocular tissue fluid levels. Make sure the BSS is hooked up to the tubing correctly and that the

FIGURE 7–13 Phaco machine (Courtesy of Advanced Medical Optics, Inc.).

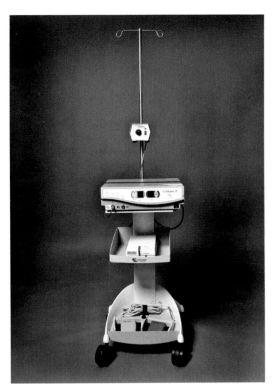

FIGURE 7–14 Coblator.

tubing is primed prior to the procedure. The level of BSS in the bottle needs to be monitored to make sure it does not run out during the procedure.

There are several types of handpieces available, which allows the surgeon to customize the surgery to the needs of the patient.

EAR NOSE THROAT MACHINES

Coblator

The coblator (see Fig. 7-14) is used for tissue destruction and coagulation during ear nose throat (ENT) procedures, most notably tonsillectomy and adenoidectomy. The tissue is removed by molecular disintegration, and the tissue bed is coagulated using bipolar energy. Most of the handpieces used with the machine have built-in suction and irrigation (saline delivery).

There are different handpieces (also called *wands*) that allow the machine to be used for the following:

- Tonsillectomy
- Adenoidectomy
- Uvulopalatoplasty
- Submucosal tissue shrinkage in the oral and nasal cavities

Straight Shot

The Xomed XPS microdissector (also known as a *straight shot*) is used for sinus surgery. Several handpieces (see Fig. 7-15) are

FIGURE 7–15 Straight shot console and handpiece.

available that allow the machine to be used for medial and lateral cutting in the frontal sinuses as well as polyp removal in the maxillary sinus. The cutting is done by a rotating blade at the tip of the handpiece.

The newer version of this system (XPS 3000) offers the option of running a high-speed otologic drill for treatment of acoustic neuroma or performance of cochleostomy. The drill burr rotates at 80,000 RPM in both forward and reverse and has a built-in water cooling system.

GYNECOLOGIAL SURGERY MACHINES

Morcellator

The morcellator is a used to cut tissue into small pieces so that it can be removed through a small opening or laparoscopic port. One of the most common uses is to make the fibroid uterus small enough to remove vaginally during vaginal hysterectomies (laparoscopic assisted or regular).

The morcellator is a single patient use device. It is plugged into a motor drive unit (power box). Like all powered devices, the morcellator should be plugged and tested prior to the start of the procedure to ensure that it is working properly. The tips of the newer power morcellators are coated with titanium nitrate to make them more resistant to dulling as they cut tissue. They have a safety guard that can be activated to shield healthy tissue from damage.

There are some manual (nonpowered) morcellators that are used to cut bone or cartilage. The manual morcellators are made of metal and are able to be resterilized.

Many types of morcellators are available for various surgical specialties: gynecology, urology (for prostate surgery), orthopedics (for bone morcellization), and general surgery (for laparoscopic procedures). Morcellators are used only on tissue masses that the surgeon is convinced are benign.

As with any device, it is imperative that all personnel in the OR be familiar with the operation and safety precautions associated with the particular morcellator in use.

Vacuum Curettage

The electric vacuum curettage (see Fig. 7-16) is used to remove endometrial tissue or products of conception during dilation and evacuation (D&E). The D&E can be performed electively or to treat conditions such as a miscarriage, missed or incomplete abortion, or retained placental tissue. This procedure is used most commonly to treat conditions occurring in the first trimester of pregnancy.

A dilation and curettage (D&C) is performed. Once the cervix is dilated, a disposable curette is attached to the vacuum aspirator suction tubing, the vacuum is activated and the uterine contents are evacuated. The machine has two collection bottles where the specimen is collected for later retrieval.

The vacuum power on the machine is adjustable. Curettes are available in a variety of diameters from 7 mm to 12 mm.

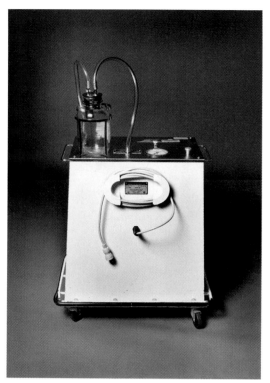

FIGURE 7–16 Vacuum curettage machine.

LIPOSUCTION

Liposuction is the surgical aspiration of excess fat for the purpose of improving body contours. The excess fat is suctioned out through the use of specially designed metal suction cannulas and an aspiration machine. Liposuction can be performed on almost any part of the body and has become one of the most commonly performed aesthetic surgeries.

The aspiration machine (see Fig. 7-17) is a high vacuum machine because fat is thick and cannot be removed from the body using regular suction. The recommended suction setting for liposuction is about −500 mm Hg and the highest suction setting on many regular suction canisters is −350 mm Hg.

Prior to skin incision, the tissue is injected with a mixture of lidocaine, epinephrine and Ringer's lactate intravenous solution. The purpose of the injection is to expand the tissue for easier insertion of the cannula, to provide hemostasis (epinephrine) and to provide local anesthesia (lidocaine). Small incisions are made, the cannula is passed under the skin and the excess fat is suctioned out.

MICROSCOPE

The microscope is commonly used in the OR for a variety of microsurgical procedures (see Fig. 7-18). Many procedures require that the surgeon be able to reattach or reanastomose tiny structures that would be hard to see with the naked eye. The microscope makes this job easier by magnifying the surgical

FIGURE 7–17 A) Aspirator. B) Liposuction cannulae.

FIGURE 7–18 Microscope.

field. A structure as fine as a hair can look like a piece of rope when magnified under a microscope.

Microscopes are used in a multitude of surgical specialties. Some examples of procedures using a microscope include the following:

- *Urology:* Vasovasotomy (reanastomosis of the vas deferens)
- *Neurosurgery:* Removal of small tumors or vascular anomalies
- *Reimplantation procedures:* Suturing of tiny nerves and blood vessels
- *Gynecological surgery:* Tubal reanastomosis
- *ENT:* Middle ear surgery

- *Eye surgery:* Vitrectomy, corneal transplant
- *Vascular:* Reanastomosis or repair of tiny blood vessels

The microscope has several components with which OR personnel need to be familiar. The lens system (see Fig. 7-19) consists of two types of lenses: *objective* and *ocular*. *Ocular lenses* are proximal lenses or eyepieces that the surgeon looks through. The ocular lens magnifies the field of view. *Objective lenses* are the distal lenses. Objective lenses provide magnification and establish the working distance from the surgical field. In order to figure out how much magnification is being used, multiply the magnification of the objective lenses by the magnification of the ocular lenses. For example:

300 (magnification of objective lens) × 10 (magnification of ocular lens) = 3000 (total magnification)

The lens system has a focus control to allow the surgeon to sharpen the view of the surgical field. The focus control may be hand operated with knobs or controlled by a foot pedal, depending on the model.

Every microscope has an illumination (lighting) system that allows for visualization of the field. This lighting system is usually made of fiberoptics and is referred to as the *coaxial illuminator*. The *paraxial illuminator* is made up of light tubes that contain bulbs and focusing lenses. This system allows light to focus as the working distance of the scope is changed.

Microscopes come equipped with a zoom lens to allow for changes in magnification of the field. These systems are operated by foot pedals, so it is important that the circulator

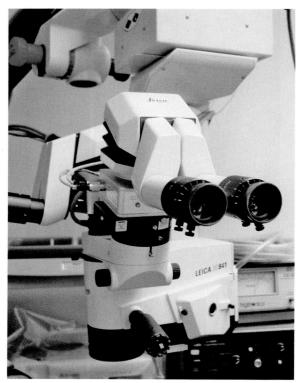

FIGURE 7–19 Lens system.

make sure that the foot pedal is within easy reach of the surgeon's foot.

One important accessory is the *beam splitter*. The beam splitter transmits the image seen by the primary ocular to the secondary (or assistant's) ocular and produces an identical image so that the assistant can see exactly what the surgeon is seeing. The beam splitter also can be used with a camera to allow the picture to be projected onto a monitor for viewing by the entire team.

Microscopes are very delicate pieces of machinery. The lenses can be easily scratched or damaged, fiberoptics can be broken or the internal components could be jarred loose or broken. Listed are tips for the handling and moving of microscopes.

ROBOTICS

Robotic surgery, once considered a technology of the distant future, is now quickly becoming routine for some procedures. Robotic equipment has been designed to enhance minimally invasive procedures. The instruments and camera are attached to the machine's robotic arms. The robotic arms are manipulated by a surgeon who is seated at a console. This allows him or her to perform the surgery without standing at the surgical field.

Robotic surgery is now an accepted way to perform several surgeries across a number of specialties. Surgical procedures in which robotics are currently being used include the following:

WATCH OUT! **Microscope Care and Handling**

- Never place your fingers on the lenses.
- Clean the lenses with a cleaner recommended by the manufacturer or with lens paper.
- Wipe down the microscope casing before and after the procedure, following your institution's procedures for equipment decontamination.
- Leave the microscope covered while it is being stored. This will help to protect the lenses from scratches as well as keep dust from collecting on the casing.
- Store the microscope with the lens caps in place.
- Check all cords and plugs for fraying. If a cord or plug is damaged, do not use the microscope. Get a replacement microscope and have biomedical engineering check the damaged one.
- When moving the microscope, secure the arm so that it cannot swing outward and hit a doorway or wall.
- Never move the microscope by holding onto it by the head. Always move it by holding onto the center of the vertical column with two hands.
- Make sure the brakes work prior to moving the microscope up to the surgical field.
- Check the focus knobs and zoom control prior to the case to make sure they are working properly.
- Balance the microscope prior to use. The manufacturer's instructions should be followed for this procedure.
- Be familiar with the operation and troubleshooting of the microscope prior to the case.

Refer to the manufacturer's instructions if you have questions.

- Radical prostatectomy, pyeloplasty, cystectomy, nephrectomy, ureteral reimplantation, donor nephrectomy, adrenalectomy (urology)
- Cholecystectomy, Nissen fundoplication, gastric bypass, splenectomy and bowel resection (general surgery)
- Hysterectomy, myomectomy (gynecology)
- Internal mammary artery mobilization and cardiac tissue ablation, mitral valve repair, endoscopic atrial septal defect closure, mammary to left anterior descending coronary artery anastomosis for cardiac revascularization with adjunctive mediastinotomy (cardiac surgery) (Adapted from www.intuitivesurgcial.com)

Robotic technology is not inexpensive (average cost >$1.5 million); therefore, advantages need to be looked at prior to investing in this technology. These advantages include the following:

- Elimination of hand tremor and cramping
- 3-D viewing of the surgical field
- Decrease in the number of surgical assistants needed; some systems have an optional fourth arm that can be

used for providing countertraction or aiding in suturing, allowing some procedures to be performed without an assistant.

- Increase in dexterity; the arm of the robot that holds the instruments can be rotated 360 degrees with 90 degrees of articulation
- Binocular optics, allowing for better depth perception
- Less fatigue for the surgeon

The robotic arms are the "working" part of the system. The instruments are attached to the arms (see Fig. 7-20), and the surgeon can position and manipulate the arms and instruments as needed to perform the surgery. The instruments are designed to work like a human wrist; they can be rotated 360 degrees and have 90 degrees of articulation. This amount of freedom of movement allows for more precision working around delicate structures.

The console (see Fig. 7-21) where the surgeon sits is designed to allow the surgeon to control the movements of the instruments and robotic arms through the use of hand controls and foot pedals. The surgeon looks into binocular lenses and is able to see a 3-D view of the surgical field.

The third component of the system is the monitor system. The monitor allows for the procedure to be viewed by all personnel in the room (see Fig. 7-22). It is also equipped to record the procedure for later viewing or to print out pictures for the patient's medical record.

Robotic surgery is quickly becoming the "cutting edge" of minimally invasive surgery. Advances in this technology are allowing surgeons in one location to view or perform surgery in another location (*telesurgery*). Robotics systems are becoming more sophisticated and capable of performing more precise procedures.

As more procedures are being performed using minimally invasive techniques, the use of robotic technology to perform

FIGURE 7-21 Surgeon console.

FIGURE 7-20 A) and B) Robotic arms and instrument.

these procedures is increasing. The increased use of this technology requires scrubbed personnel and circulators to be familiar with the technology, how to set up the equipment and attach the instruments and how to troubleshoot the equipment. Like any technology, there are limitations. As with any minimally invasive procedure, the OR personnel must to be able to convert to an "open" procedure if necessary. Personnel must also be ready to take over and finish the procedure manually if the robotics equipment malfunctions.

FIGURE 7–22 Monitor cart.

 Surgical Session Review

1) An ICP monitor measures pressure within the:
   a. chest
   b. cranium
   c. carpals
   d. coronaries

2) Phacoemulsification is used to remove:
   a. cataracts
   b. wrinkles
   c. chalazions
   d. vitreous humor

3) The suction pressure needed to remove fat during liposuction is about:
   a. −200 mm Hg
   b. −300 mm Hg
   c. −350 mm Hg
   d. −500 mm Hg

4) A scleral buckle procedure is used to treat:
   a. corneal abrasion
   b. glaucoma
   c. retinal detachment
   d. sties

5) Trichiasis is another name for an ingrown:
   a. toenail
   b. fingernail
   c. abscess
   d. eyelash

6) One example of a surgical robotic system is the:
   a. DeNali
   b. daVinci
   c. DeNero
   d. DeTrussor

7) Cryotherapy uses _____ to destroy tissue.
   a. heat
   b. electricity
   c. cold
   d. ultrasound

8) Diathermy uses _____ to destroy tissue.
   a. heat
   b. electricity
   c. cold
   d. ultrasound

9) A vacuum curettage machine would be used during which of the following procedures?
   a. hysterectomy
   b. oophorectomy
   c. D&E
   d. cerclage

10) The cardiopulmonary bypass machine is operated by a:
   a. surgeon
   b. nurse
   c. surgical technologist
   d. perfusionist

11) In which of the following procedures would cardiopulmonary bypass definitely *not* be used:
   a. repair of tetralogy of Fallot
   b. heart transplant
   c. aortofemoral bypass graft
   d. CABG

12) The straight shot device is used for surgery of the:
   a. hand
   b. foot
   c. back
   d. sinuses

13) A coblator is used most commonly for a:
   a. coronary bypass graft
   b. cerclage
   c. tonsillectomy
   d. adenoma removal

14) The eyepiece of a microscope is the _____ lens.
   a. objective
   b. ocular
   c. ophthalmic
   d. oculomotor

15) Examples of bone implants include all of the following *except*:
   a. staple
   b. cancellous screw
   c. fiberglass cast
   d. femoral nail

16) Which statement is *false* regarding handling of implants:
   a. handle as little as possible
   b. always measure any screw prior to handing it to the surgeon
   c. implants may be reused
   d. do not use any implant that has been damaged

17) The proper order for the steps for screw insertion is:
   a. measure, drill, tap, screw
   b. tap, measure, drill, screw
   c. drill, measure, tap, screw
   d. drill, tap, measure, screw

18) A bone tap is used to:
   a. create ridges for the screw to follow
   b. determine the length of screw needed
   c. screw the plate to the bone
   d. drill the hole for the screw

19) A CUSA or Sonopet machine is used for:
   a. excising abdominal tumors
   b. excising brain tumors
   c. excising bone tumors
   d. excising breast tumors

20) Which of the following is *not* an advantage of robotic surgery?
   a. hand tremors are minimized or eliminated
   b. increased dexterity for instrument manipulation
   c. decreased cost of machinery
   d. improved depth perception due to binocular optics

CHAPTER 8
Anesthesia Supplies and Equipment

TYPES OF ANESTHESIA

The word *anesthesia* comes from the Greek *anaisthesis* meaning "without sensation." Anesthesia allows us to perform surgery on patients without them feeling pain and, in most cases, recalling the events of the operating room (OR).

In today's surgical world, there are several types of anesthesia available: general, regional blocks (i.e., spinal, epidural and nerve blocks), monitored anesthesia care (MAC) and local. Depending on what type of surgery is being performed, the patient may have a choice of the type of anesthetic being used.

This chapter contains a brief description of each type of anesthesia, the surgery for which it is usually used, common side effects and Watch Out! boxes. Pay particular attention to the Watch Out! boxes because they are listings of what you need to look for or report if you are the person assisting the anesthesia care provider during the administration of the anesthetic.

General Anesthesia

Description
Commonly described by patients as "going off to sleep," general anesthesia consists of four components: heavy sedation (alteration of consciousness), muscle relaxation, loss of response to pain and lack of recall of events while under anesthesia. There is not one single medication that produces an adequate level of all four of these components; therefore, the anesthesia provider must use a combination of medications (usually given by the inhalation or intravenous [IV] routes) to achieve optimum results.

Stages of General Anesthesia
There are four stages to general anesthesia: induction, maintenance, emergence and recovery.

Induction Phase: During the induction phase, the patient goes from a state of consciousness to a state of unconsciousness. His or her reflexes also are depressed. Respiratory depression may occur. **Maintenance of airway is crucial during this phase!**

Cricoid pressure (also known as *Sellick's maneuver*) is performed to reduce the risk of aspiration or help the anesthesia provider visualize the vocal cords. Firm pressure is applied to the cricoid cartilage using the thumb and index finger in a V formation (see Fig. 8-1). This causes the esophagus to be occluded between the cricoid cartilage and the lower cervical vertebrae, thus decreasing the chance of aspiration. Applying pressure to the cartilage can also help to visualize the cords, especially if the patient's anatomy is less than optimal, thus

making intubation easier. When applying cricoid pressure, *do not release the pressure until instructed to do so by the anesthesia care provider.*

Maintenance: The second phase of anesthesia is maintenance of the anesthetic. It is during this phase that the surgical procedure takes place. The patient is constantly monitored for homeostasis of all vital functions, and the anesthesia care provider adjusts the anesthetic levels accordingly.

WATCH OUT! | **Induction Phase**

- Another trained person, other than the anesthesia provider, should be positioned by the patient's side near the head of the bed during induction to help, as needed.

- Personnel helping anesthesia should have the skill and knowledge to maintain the patient's airway, if need be.

- If the anesthesia provider is using an endotracheal tube, the person assisting should hold the tube and be ready to hand it to the anesthesia provider as soon as he or she visualizes the vocal cords.

- If the provider is using a stylet to intubate, pull the stylet when asked; be careful not to pull too hard or you might dislodge the tube.

- If you are providing cricoid pressure (see text for description), do not release pressure until instructed to do so by the anesthesia provider.

- Hearing is the last sense to leave the patient during induction. *Talking and noise should be kept to an absolute minimum; be careful what you say!*

FIGURE 8-1 Cricoid pressure being held on a manikin's neck.

Maintenance Phase

- The circulator needs to be aware of what is going on with the anesthesia care provider. Increased activity "behind the screen" could indicate a change in patient condition. Always keep an eye and ear out and be ready to respond if help is needed.

- Scrubbed personnel need to keep track of the amount of irrigating fluid used and report that number to the anesthesia provider. This is an important step in estimating blood loss.

- Scrubbed personnel need to tell the anesthesia provider when they are about to irrigate with large amounts of fluid. The anesthesia provider needs to be aware of this extensive irrigation so that he or she will not think a large amount of bleeding has suddenly occurred.

- When local anesthetic is used during a procedure, scrubbed personnel need to keep track of the amount injected. The amount, type and strength of local anesthetic used needs to be reported to the anesthesia care provider.

Emergence: Emergence is the third phase of general anesthesia. This phase occurs as the surgical procedure is finishing. The goal is to have the patient as awake as possible at the end of the procedure. Monitoring the patient's ability to resume breathing on his or her own and restoring a gag reflex are the focus during emergence. The patient is usually extubated, if necessary. A major concern during this phase is the risk of laryngospasm or bronchospasm, which can lead to airway obstruction. The airway must be monitored closely.

Recovery: The last phase of general anesthesia is recovery. In this phase, the patient returns to his or her optimal level of consciousness. This phase begins in the OR, continues in the PACU and may continue through discharge. Patients are closely monitored in the OR and PACU for signs of increasing levels of consciousness and function.

Emergence Phase

- Another trained person, other than the anesthesia provider, should be positioned by the patient's side near the head of the bed during emergence to help as needed.

- Personnel helping anesthesia should have the skill and knowledge to maintain the patient's airway if need be.

- Hearing is often the first sense to return during emergence. *Keep noise to an absolute minimum and be careful what is said!*

- Be prepared to assist if needed after extubation. In rare cases, the patient may need to be reintubated.

- Have oxygen ready for transport to the post-anesthesia care unit (PACU). (Make sure you have checked the amount of oxygen in the tank prior to the end of the case!)

Procedures Performed Under General Anesthesia

Any surgical procedure can be performed while the patient is under general anesthesia. The anesthesia care provider, along with the patient and surgeon, decide if the patient is a candidate for general anesthesia.

Advantages
- Medication dosages can be adjusted as needed.
- Muscle relaxation can be achieved, making for easier visualization within the surgical field.
- Rate and depth of respiration can be controlled.
- Patient is usually unaware of what goes on intraoperatively.

Disadvantages
- A small percentage of patients are aware of intraoperative events.
- General anesthesia is not for everyone. If the patient has many co-morbidities, then he or she may not be a good candidate to undergo general anesthesia.
- Risk of aspiration is greatest during the induction and emergence phases.
- Risk of laryngospasm or bronchospasm is real.
- Risk of malignant hyperthermia is real, although rare, as anesthesia personnel screen patients preoperatively for risk of malignant hyperthermia.
- There is an increased chance of postoperative nausea and vomiting.
- There is an increased chance of postoperative pain when compared with regional anesthesia.

Regional Anesthesia

Spinal Anesthesia

To perform a spinal block, the anesthesia care provider injects an anesthetic agent into the subarachnoid space using a spinal needle inserted into an intervertebral space in the lower lumbar area. The patient experiences loss of sensation below the diaphragm.

Procedures Performed Under Spinal Anesthesia

Spinal anesthesia can be used for procedures below the waist. It is most commonly used for orthopedic procedures on the lower limbs (e.g., total knee arthroplasty, total hip arthroplasty), genitourinary procedures and gynecological procedures.

Advantages
- Patients remain conscious and in control of their own airways.
- Patients can receive sedation that is titrated to their desired levels of consciousness during the procedure.
- Patients suffer less systemic effects with spinal anesthesia than with general anesthesia; therefore, spinal anesthesia may be a less risky choice of anesthetic for those with multiple co-morbidities.

WATCH OUT! Spinal Anesthesia

- Hypotension (sudden drop in blood pressure) is a major risk with spinal anesthesia. The person assisting the anesthesia care provider must keep an eye on the blood pressure monitor and report a drop of more than 20 systolic to the anesthesia provider immediately. Often, the anesthesia provider's back is to the monitors while inserting the spinal needle; therefore, it is up to the person assisting to watch for hypotension. Continuous monitoring of vital signs is necessary.

- There is a small chance that the spinal block could move upward thereby blocking the diaphragm and accessory respiratory muscles. The person assisting the anesthesia care provider needs to monitor the patient for signs of difficulty breathing or respiratory distress.

- Proper positioning of the patient before needle insertion is important. A spinal anesthetic can be administered with the patient either lying on his or her side or sitting up and leaning forward (this is usually the anesthesia provider's preference). The person assisting needs to help the patient into the proper position and help the patient maintain that position throughout the procedure; this may require holding the patient in position, especially if he or she has been sedated.

- *Remember:* Watch what is said in the room. The patient is awake!

- Patients do not experience the sore throat or hoarseness postoperatively that an endotracheal tube (ETT) can cause.
- Produces bowel contraction, which can facilitate exposure during surgery of the abdomen or pelvis.
- Produces muscle relaxation, making retraction easier.

Disadvantages
- Hypotension! Monitor the patient for signs of decreased blood pressure.
- The spinal block could travel upward and block the muscles necessary for respiration. Monitor the patient for signs of difficulty breathing.
- In a small percentage of cases, the spinal anesthetic is not effective and the patient must be given a general anesthetic.
- The dosage of medication cannot be titrated. Once it is given, it cannot be adjusted.
- It is possible for the patient to experience a spinal headache postoperatively.
- The patient could possibly develop temporary or permanent paraesthesia or paralysis (very rare).
- Spinal anesthesia cannot be used for procedures of long duration. The length of time you get depends on the anesthetic agent that is used.

Epidural Anesthesia
Epidural anesthesia is accomplished by the anesthesia care provider injecting an anesthetic agent into the epidural space that surrounds the dural sac. The anesthetic agent is absorbed slowly through the dura mater into the cerebrospinal fluid.

WATCH OUT! Epidural Anesthesia

- The agent is more slowly absorbed; therefore, hypotension develops more slowly than with a spinal block, making it easier to treat.

- Accidental puncture of the dura during needle insertion could result in total spinal anesthesia. Signs of total spinal anesthesia include bradycardia, respiratory paralysis and vasodilation.

- Continuous monitoring of vital signs is necessary during insertion of an epidural.

- *Remember:* Watch what is said in the room; the patient is awake!

Epidural anesthesia can be a single shot of anesthetic agent or, more commonly, a small catheter is inserted into the back and an intermittent or continuous drip of medication is administered through the catheter to provide ongoing pain control.

Procedures Performed Under Epidural Anesthesia
Epidural anesthesia is commonly used for procedures of the rectum and pelvis (e.g., obstetrical, gynecological and urological). It can be used for intraoperative and postoperative pain control or, in some cases, control of intractable pain.

Advantages
- Medication dosage can be titrated.
- When the need is no longer there, the catheter can be removed.
- Postoperative pain control can be achieved yet the patient is able to walk and move about.
- The medication pump delivering the agent can be programmed to allow the patient to deliver supplemental doses of medication, as needed.
- The patient remains conscious and cooperative (important during labor).
- Patient remains in control of his or her own airway.

Disadvantages
- Hypotension can result, although more slowly than with a spinal block.
- In rare cases, the epidural may not be effective, necessitating a switch to another type of anesthetic.
- Accidental puncture of the dura during the insertion could result in total spinal anesthesia leading to respiratory paralysis and bradycardia.

Combined Spinal/Epidural Anesthesia

Description
An epidural needle is passed into the epidural space in the usual manner. A spinal needle is passed through the epidural needle until the dura is pierced. Medication is injected into the subarachnoid space. The spinal needle is removed and an epidural catheter is placed into the epidural space.

Combined Spinal/Epidural Anesthesia

- Same as for epidural and spinal anesthesia.

- Some patients experience pruritus (itching) after injection of the narcotic.

- *Remember:* Watch what is said in the room; the patient is awake!

Procedures Performed Under Spinal/Epidural Anesthesia

Combined spinal/epidural anesthesia is commonly used for obstetrical procedures or labor pain relief. This technique can also be used for surgical procedures that have extended surgery times.

Advantages

- Spinal/epidural anesthesia provides immediate benefits from the spinal injection, but use of the epidural catheter allows for continued anesthesia.
- This type of anesthesia offers less motor block than spinal anesthesia alone.
- Patient remains conscious and cooperative, which is important during labor.
- Patient remains in control of his or her own airway.

Disadvantages

- Hypotension! Monitor the patient for signs of decreased blood pressure.
- There is the potential for the patient to experience a spinal headache postoperatively.
- The patient could potentially develop temporary or permanent paraesthesia or paralysis (very rare).

Nerve Block

Nerve blocks are another option for regional anesthesia. The anesthesia care provider injects an anesthetic agent into either a large peripheral nerve or the area of a *major nerve plexus* (a large bundle or group of nerves). This type of anesthesia allows for temporary loss of sensation to the area innovated by the nerve or plexus.

Nerve Blocks

- Most of the major nerves run near major arteries. If the medication is accidently injected into the artery, anesthetic overdose could occur. The patient's vital signs should be monitored closely throughout the procedure.

- The anesthesia care provider may ask the person assisting him or her to inject the medication once the correct spot is found. The assistant should aspirate (pull back slightly on the plunger) then inject 5 to 10 cc of the medication slowly. The assistant should aspirate every 5 to 10 cc until the anesthetic is injected.

- *Remember:* Watch what is said in the room; the patient is awake!

Procedures Performed Under Nerve Block

Nerve blocks are commonly used for procedures on the arm or leg. In addition to intraoperative anesthesia, nerve blocks help control postoperative pain (many agents last 18 to 24 hours). In selected cases, a nerve block can be used to control intractable pain (e.g., injection of the intercostal nerves to control rib pain).

Advantages

- Nerve block anesthesia can be given to a specific area only, without the systemic impact of a general or spinal anesthetic.
- Nerve blocks allow analgesia to continue into the postoperative period.
- The duration of the block is medication-specific, allowing it to be tailored to the specific needs of the patient and/or procedure.
- Patient is conscious and in control of his or her own airway
- Nerve blocks can be combined with other types of anesthesia (e.g., general).

Disadvantages

- Anesthetic overdose could occur if a major artery is accidently injected, causing seizures or cardiac arrest.

Bier Block

A Bier block is a regional block of the distal end of an upper extremity. A tourniquet is placed on the upper arm, and the anesthetic is injected intravenously at an area close to the surgical site. The limb is exsanguinated using an Esmarch bandage, and the proximal tourniquet is inflated to about 100 mm Hg above the patient's systolic blood pressure. The tourniquet remains inflated throughout the procedure to prevent the anesthetic agent from being redistributed from the area.

Procedures Performed Under Bier Blocks

Procedures of the distal upper extremity that are less then 1 hour in duration (e.g., closed reduction of a Colles fracture)

Advantages

- Bier block is a short-acting, localized anesthesia without systemic impact.

Bier Block

- If the tourniquet fails or the tourniquet is released too rapidly at the end of the procedure, the patient may experience systemic administration of the medication. Systemic administration can adversely affect the cardiovascular system, causing sudden changes in heart rate and blood pressure. The patient's vital signs should be closely monitored throughout the injection, surgical procedure and release of the tourniquet.

- *Remember:* Watch what is said in the room; the patient is awake!

- It has a short recovery time after the procedure.
- Patient is conscious and in control of his or her own airway.

Disadvantages

- It has limited uses (distal upper extremity procedures of short duration).
- Patient could experience adverse cardiovascular effects due to systemic administration of the medication.

Monitored Anesthesia Care

The patient receives sedatives, analgesics or amnesics to make him or her less aware of intraoperative events. This is done in conjunction with a local anesthetic at the surgical site.

Procedures Performed Under Monitored Anesthesia Care

Monitored anesthesia care (MAC) can be used for procedures that can be done using local anesthesia, when the patient wants some sedation.

Advantages

- MAC can be used for patients with complex medical problems who are undergoing procedures requiring only local anesthesia
- It has fewer systemic effects than other types of anesthesia.
- Medication dosages can be titrated.
- There is a short recovery time after the procedure.
- Patient is conscious and in control of his or her own airway.

Disadvantages

- MAC cannot be used for complex procedures.
- Patient must be able to be cooperative (e.g., not moving the area the surgeon is working on).

Local Anesthesia

Local anesthesia is produced when the surgeon injects an anesthetic agent into the tissue surrounding the operative site. This

> **WATCH OUT!** **Monitored Anesthesia Care**
>
> - Supplemental oxygen should be available.
> - The patient's vital signs (especially respiratory status) and level of consciousness need to be closely monitored; usually this is done by the anesthesia care provider, but the circulator must be aware of what is happening.
> - Scrubbed personnel need to keep track of the amount of local anesthetic injected at the surgical site. They need to the anesthesia care provider the type, strength and amount of local used.
> - *Remember:* Watch what is said in the room; the patient is awake!

> **WATCH OUT!** **Local Anesthesia: Topical Anesthesia**
>
> - Depending on institution policy, if the patient is undergoing only local anesthesia, a registered nurse (RN) may be monitoring the patient's vital signs intraoperatively. The RN should NOT be the same nurse who is performing the circulating duties; a dedicated nurse should be assigned to monitor the patient.
> - Supplemental oxygen should be available.
> - If sedation (e.g., Versed) is being used, the institution's policy for conscious sedation must be followed.
> - Scrubbed personnel need to keep track of the amount of local anesthetic injected at the surgical site and report to the person monitoring the patient the type, strength and amount of local used.
> - *Remember:* Watch what is said in the room; the patient is awake!

produces a small, localized area of anesthesia/analgesia at the operative site. The length of the anesthesia/analgesia depends on the agent used.

Procedures Performed Under Local Anesthesia

Local anesthesia can be used for simple or short procedures (e.g., wound suturing, pacemaker insertion, chest tube insertion and removal of small skin lesions). Some surgeons perform breast biopsy and hernia repairs using local anesthesia.

Advantages

- Local anesthesia can be used for patients with complex medical problems who are undergoing procedures requiring only local anesthesia.
- Local anesthesia has fewer systemic effects than other types of anesthesia.
- There is a short recovery time after the procedure than when general anesthesia is used.
- Patient is conscious and in control of his or her own airway.
- Surgeon can regulate the amount of medication that the patient receives based on the patient's needs.

Disadvantages

- Cannot be used for complex procedures.
- Patient must be able to be cooperative (e.g., not moving the area the surgeon is working on).
- May require another RN to be assigned to monitor the patient, depending on institution policy.

Topical Anesthesia

Topical anesthesia is produced by instilling or swabbing a local anesthetic agent onto mucous membranes or tissue.

Procedures Performed Under Topical Anesthesia

Topical anesthesia can be used for minor, short-duration procedures of the mucous membranes or skin (e.g., skin tag removal,

---

WATCH OUT! | **Topical Anesthesia**

- Observe the patient for signs of allergic reaction to the medication.

- Keep track of the amount, type and strength of medication and chart on the patient's chart.

- *Remember:* Watch what is said in the room; the patient is awake!

---

throat endoscopy and IV insertion) or as a supplement to other anesthesia (e.g., cocaine in nasal procedures). Topical anesthesia is often used for cataract surgery.

Advantages
- Topical anesthesia requires a very short recovery time.
- There are fewer systemic effects following topical than other types of anesthesia.
- Patient is conscious and in control of his or her own airway.

Disadvantages
- Topical anesthesia cannot be used for complex procedures.
- Patient must be able to be cooperative (e.g., not moving the area the surgeon is working on).

AIRWAYS

When a patient can no longer adequately maintain a patent airway independently, several types of adjuncts can be used. The type of airway chosen depends on the situation: why the person can no longer maintain his or her own airway, how long the surgical procedure is expected to last or if the person is expected to need ventilatory support postoperatively. This section covers oral and nasal airways, laryngeal mask airways (LMAs), and several types of ETTs.

Oral Airways

An oral airway is a curved piece of rigid plastic with an opening through the middle or along the sides (see Fig. 8-2). It can help to establish or maintain a patent airway in an unconscious patient, or it can be inserted in the mouth to keep the patient from biting down on the ETT.

The oral airway works by lifting the tongue forward to keep it from obstructing the pharynx. This type of airway is to be used only in an unconscious patient without a gag reflex. If the patient has a gag reflex, insertion of an oral airway could lead to gagging, vomiting or laryngospasm.

Oral airways do not require any special equipment to insert. The airway is inserted into the mouth with the curve facing the roof of the mouth, and then the airway is rotated 180 degrees as you move it toward the back of the oral cavity. The airway tip should come to rest at the front of the pharynx, just behind the back of the tongue, with the phalange of the airway between

FIGURE 8-2 Oral airway.

the patient's lips. The curve of the airway is resting on the tongue, holding it down and keeping the passage to the pharynx open. An alternative method of inserting an oral airway is to depress the tongue with a tongue blade and insert the airway with the tip facing the floor of the mouth.

Oral airways are available in a variety of sizes to fit anyone from a newborn (size 000 or 30-mm long) to a large adult (size 6 or 120-mm long). To approximate the correct size for your patient, place the phalange of the airway at the base of the patient's ear lobe and lay the airway diagonally across the cheek to the corner of the patient's mouth (on the same side of the face). The tip of the airway should reach the corner of the mouth without overlap (see Fig. 8-3). If the airway overlaps the lips, the airway is too large; if it doesn't reach the corner of the mouth, the airway is too small.

Nasal Airways

Unlike the oral airway, nasal airways can be used to help maintain an airway in a patient who still has a gag reflex (see Fig. 8-4). The nasal airway is a soft hollow tube with a phalange at one end to prevent it from slipping all the way into

FIGURE 8-3 Correctly sized airway next to manikin's face.

FIGURE 8-4 Nasal airway.

the nasal cavity. It rests in the nasopharynx and does not go down far enough into the throat to trigger the gag reflex.

To insert the airway, lubricate it with water-soluble lubricant and insert it into the nares, advancing along the floor of the nasal passage and into the nasopharynx. Nasal airways come in a variety of diameters ranging from 12 Fr to 36 Fr.

Nasal airways could cause *epistaxis* (nasal bleeding) and should not be used in a patient who is on anticoagulants. They should also not be used in children with prominent adenoids or in a patient with a basilar skull fracture.

Laryngeal Mask Airway

The LMA consists of a wide tube with a 15-mm connector at one end that connects to an anesthesia breathing circuit and an elliptical inflatable cuff at the other end that, when inflated, sits in the laryngopharynx. There are three fenestrations in the cuff to allow for ventilation of the patient (see Fig. 8-5). The cuff is inflated through a pilot tube.

The LMA is becoming increasingly popular as a device to deliver anesthetics for general anesthesia. The LMA does not go through or below the vocal cords and, when properly used, can have less complications then an ETT.

Not all general anesthesia patients are candidates for the use of an LMA. The LMA should not be used in patients with a full stomach or hiatal hernia, patients with pharyngeal pathology (e.g., abscess, tumor or obstruction), patients undergoing lengthy procedures or patients requiring high peak inspiratory pressures.

The LMA comes in both re-sterilizable and disposable types. Sizes range from size 2 (infant) to size 6 (large adult).

In addition to providing a patent airway, facilitating ventilation and providing a conduit to deliver anesthetic gases, a special type of LMA can be used to help facilitate placement of an ETT in a patient with a difficult airway. This type of LMA is known as a *Fastrach LMA* (see Fig. 8-6).

Endotracheal Tubes

The ETT or endotracheal tube (also known as an ET or a TT) is a tube used to provide a patent airway, deliver anesthetic gases, control ventilation and prevent aspiration during general anesthesia. When you hear about a patient "being intubated," it is generally referring to the placement of an ETT.

ETTs come either *cuffed*, meaning that they have an inflatable balloon on one end that holds them in place in the trachea, or *uncuffed*, which means there is not an inflatable balloon on the end (see Fig. 8-7). Although there are exceptions, generally uncuffed tubes are used in small children (to avoid pressure injury to the trachea from the balloon), and cuffed tubes are used in older children and adults.

ETTs come in sizes ranging from 2.5 (infant) though 9.0 (large adult). ETTs are single patient use and cannot be re-sterilized.

To insert an ETT, the anesthesia care provider uses a laryngoscope. The laryngoscope consists of a handle with an electrical contact onto which a blade with a light bulb is attached. The lighted blade is inserted into the larynx, allowing the anesthesia care provider to examine the larynx and visualize the vocal cords.

There are two different types of blades that can be attached to the laryngoscope. The Macintosh (or Mac) blade is curved,

FIGURE 8-5 LMA.

FIGURE 8-6 Fastrach LMA.

FIGURE 8–7 Cuffed and uncuffed ETT.

FIGURE 8–8 Laryngoscope handle along with a Miller and a Mac blade.

WATCH OUT!	Troubleshooting the Laryngoscope

If the light on the laryngoscope is dim or doesn't work, consider the following:

- Does the handle need new batteries?

- If it is a rechargeable handle, does it need to be plugged into a socket to recharge? In this case, you need to get another handle to use now.

- Is the electrical contact on the top of the handle tight? If it has come loose, you will not get good contact between the blade and the handle.

- Is the light bulb on the blade screwed into the socket tightly?

- Does the light bulb on the blade need to be replaced?

and the Miller is straight (see Fig. 8-8). Which type of blade the anesthesia care provider uses depends on patient anatomy and, to some degree, personal preference.

As with the ETTs, laryngoscope blades come in a range of sizes from infant/small child (size 0) to large adult (size 4). Laryngoscope handles come in pediatric and adult sizes.

Specialty Endotracheal Tubes

Right-Angle Endotracheal Tubes: In addition to regular ETTs, there are several tubes designed for specific purposes. The right-angle ETT (see Fig. 8-9) is specially designed for use in ear nose throat and ophthalmic surgery. This tube has a preformed right-angle bend at the level of the teeth that allows it to exit the mouth away from the surgical field.

Laser Surgery Endotracheal Tubes: Due to the possible danger of fire during laser surgery of the face and neck if a conventional ETT is used, a specially designed laser surgery ETT may be necessary. These tubes laser strikes. The cuff of the tube should be inflated with saline mixed with methylene blue to signal if the cuff is hit with the laser and ruptures (see Fig. 8-10).

Double-Lumen Bronchial Tubes: The last type of specialty ETT (see Fig. 8-11) I want to cover is the double-lumen bronchial

FIGURE 8–9 Right-angle ETT.

FIGURE 8–10 Laser ETT.

FIGURE 8–11 Double-lumen ETT.

tube. This type of tube is used for thoracic surgery. The advantage to this tube is that it allows the anesthesia care provider to ventilate one lung at a time or both together and allows suctioning of either lung.

Tracheotomy Tubes

Tracheotomy tubes are airways that are specially designed to fit inside a tracheostomy stoma in order to keep it open and provide a patent airway. A tracheostomy (also called a *tracheotomy*) can be temporary or permanent, depending on the need of the patient. It can be done as an emergency procedure or as an elective procedure. Acute upper airway obstruction is the most common reason for an emergency tracheostomy. Conditions causing upper airway obstruction include tumor, infection, foreign body, congenital or neurological conditions and trauma. Electively, a tracheostomy is often performed for patients who require long-term ventilator support or have a condition causing chronic upper airway obstruction.

Tracheotomy tubes are available cuffed (with a balloon) or uncuffed (see Fig. 8-12). Cuffed tracheotomy tubes are used for adults, especially those on ventilators. When the patient is on a ventilator, the cuff must be inflated to prevent air from leaking out around the tube. The cuff may also help prevent saliva or other secretions from entering the lungs. Like ETTs, the uncuffed tracheotomy tubes are generally used on children. Uncuffed tracheotomy tubes also can be used in adults who do not require ventilatory support.

Tracheotomy tubes consist of an outer tube and an obturator (introducer). Many tracheotomy tubes also have a removable inner cannula (see Fig. 8-13). The inner cannula slides inside the outer tube and can be removed for ease of cleaning or to unblock the tube if it becomes plugged with mucus.

Tracheotomy tubes are available in a variety of styles, can be either metal or plastic and come with outer diameter sizes ranging from 4 mm (infant) to 13 mm (large adult).

SUPPLEMENTAL OXYGEN

Oxygen is one of the most important gases in our environment. Without it, our cells could not function and we would die. We need a constant supply of oxygen, usually from the air we breathe. There are people whose bodies cannot supply their cells with adequate oxygen from breathing, commonly due to lung or heart disease, who need an additional oxygen source, usually a portable or fixed oxygen tank.

Even if we are breathing adequately, there are times that additional oxygen is needed. Preoperatively or intraoperatively, regional or MAC medication may be given to help patients relax, but it can make them drowsy, less apt to take deep breaths and in need of an additional source of oxygen. Prior to induction of general anesthetic, patients are asked to breathe oxygen to fill their lungs and give them an oxygen reserve. Oxygen is given (along with the gases) during general anesthetic to keep the body cells functioning properly. Postoperatively, oxygen is given to help the patient wake up from anesthesia as well as to help combat the effects of the anesthetics and narcotics.

There are several devices that can be used to deliver supplemental oxygen: nasal cannulas, reservoir and nonreservoir masks, bag-valve-mask devices and nebulizers. These devices and their use are covered in this section.

FIGURE 8–12 Cuffed and uncuffed tracheotomy tubes.

FIGURE 8–13 Parts of a tracheotomy tube.

WATCH OUT! **Oxygen is a Medication**

Because oxygen is used so commonly in the OR environment, we tend to forget that it is a *medication*, requiring a doctor's (or certified registered nurse anesthetist's) order for its use. Many institutions have standing orders for the use of oxygen. Be sure to check your institution's policies and procedures.

Nasal Cannula

A nasal cannula, also called *nasal prongs,* consists of two soft plastic tubes that are inserted into the patient's nostrils (see Fig. 8-14). These tubes are attached to a loop of narrow plastic hose that is looped around the patient's ears and under his or her chin to keep the prongs in place. The hose is attached to an oxygen supply (tank or wall source).

A nasal cannula delivers a lower concentration of oxygen (23% to 35%) than an oxygen mask. It is used for those patients requiring smaller amounts of supplemental oxygen (e.g., patients who have been medicated and are drowsy). The oxygen flow is generally set at 1 to 4 L/minute (*Note:* Be sure to check the order for flow setting).

Most patients tolerate a nasal cannula well, even those who are claustrophobic, because it does not cover the mouth and nose like an oxygen mask does. The nasal prongs can be irritating, mostly because the oxygen is not humidified and it dries out the mucous membranes of the nostrils.

Nasal cannulas are available in several styles and in adult and pediatric sizes.

Nonreservoir Mask

The nonreservoir or "simple" oxygen mask is a lightweight, plastic, somewhat triangle shaped device designed to cover the patient's mouth and nose (see Fig. 8-15). The mask is placed on the patient's face with the pointed end over the top of the patient's nose and the rounded end below the patient's mouth. It is attached to the patient's head using an elastic strap to secure it in place. The hose is attached to an oxygen supply (tank or wall source).

Simple masks can deliver oxygen concentrations of 30% to 45% with a flow rate of 5 to 6 L/minute and 40% to 60% with a flow rate of 7 to 8 L/minute. These masks should be used for patients requiring higher oxygen concentrations than can be delivered by nasal cannulas but who are expected to need the oxygen for short-term use (e.g., patients in the PACU waking up from anesthesia). These devices are not for use in patients who are profoundly hypoxic or tachypnic.

Nonreservoir masks are available in adult and pediatric sizes.

Reservoir Mask

The reservoir mask is an oxygen mask that has a built-in gas reservoir. There are two types: partial rebreathing mask and nonrebreathing mask. The differences are in the valves in the mask and between the mask and bag. Reservoir masks are the delivery device of choice for patients needing high concentrations of oxygen for short periods of time; that is, those who may have significant hypoxemia but are breathing relatively normally (e.g., myocardial infarction or trauma patients).

The partial rebreathing mask has a reservoir where "part" (thus the phrase *partial rebreathing*) of the patient's expired gas volume fills the reservoir bag (see Fig. 8-16). The expired gas mixes with the fresh gas (oxygen). Usually, this expired gas is mostly dead space and does not result in the patient rebreathing a significant amount of carbon dioxide. The mixing of the fresh and expired gases can potentially conserve oxygen use. Oxygen concentrations of 35% to 60% can be obtained with a flow rate of 7 to 10 L/minute.

WATCH OUT! **Simple Oxygen Mask**

The body of the mask acts as a reservoir for oxygen and expired carbon dioxide. In order for the patient to avoid rebreathing his or her own carbon dioxide, a *minimum* flow rate of 5 L/minute is required when using a simple mask.

FIGURE 8–14 Nasal cannula.

FIGURE 8–15 Nonreservoir mask.

FIGURE 8-16 Partial rebreather mask.

FIGURE 8-17 Self-inflating bag.

WATCH OUT! **Reservoir Mask**

One important factor in determining the oxygen concentration of any mask is that it fits the face properly. The mask should completely cover the mouth and nose and fit snuggly against the face without large gaps.

The nonrebreathing mask (see Fig. 8-16) has a flap-type valve between the mask and bag (reservoir) and over at least one of the mask's side ports (exhalation port). The valve between the bag and reservoir prevents expired air from entering the mask (and being rebreathed) while the valve over the side port limits the amount of room air that can enter the mask. Oxygen concentrations of 100% can be obtained with a flow rate of 15 L/minute.

Reservoir masks are available in adult in pediatric sizes. To work properly, these types of masks must be used with a flow rate of at least 7 L/minute.

Bag-Valve-Mask Device

Commonly referred to as a *BVM device,* the bag-valve-mask is used to provide ventilation to the patient who is unable to breathe (or breathe adequately) on his or her own. There are two types of devices: the anesthesia bag and the disposable self-inflating "Ambu"-type bag (see Fig. 8-17).

The anesthesia bag is a non–self-inflating bag that requires a continuous oxygen source to keep the reservoir (bag) inflated. These systems have adjustable valves to allow for the regulation of oxygen flow in response to changing breathing patterns or demands. The bags on these systems should not be allowed to deflate substantially; therefore, oxygen flow to the system should be kept relatively high (although the bag should not be allowed to overinflate either).

The self-inflating bags are used most often when a patient is in respiratory arrest or when a patient who cannot adequately breathe is being transported to another area such as a PACU or intensive care unit. In order to ventilate the patient,

the bag is attached to a mask or ETT, the bag is squeezed (just hard enough to make the chest rise) and then the bag is released.

Caution: Unlike the anesthesia bag that deflates if the flow of oxygen is inadequate (a visual sign that something is wrong), these bags do not look any different. The equipment needs to be checked to make sure that the hose is attached to the oxygen source, that the oxygen source is turned on and that there is an adequate flow rate (15 L/minute).

Nebulizers

Nebulizers can be used to deliver moistened (mist) oxygen therapy or medications to patients. These devices are adjustable to allow for the delivery of a variety of oxygen concentrations, depending on patient need. One common use for these devices in the surgical setting is post-intubation in the PACU because of the aerosol (mist) properties that help to moisten the airway (see Fig. 8-18).

Nebulizers used for mist therapy come in a variety of devices including face tents, tracheostomy collars or T pieces (that fit on ETTs). Depending on the liter flow of gas and the valve adjustment, these devices can deliver oxygen concentrations of 24% to 100%.

Nebulizers that are used for medication administration are handheld. The medication and a small amount of saline are added to the chamber of the nebulizer and oxygen flow is turned on. The medication is converted to an aerosol form

WATCH OUT! **Nebulizer Treatments**

When nebulizers are used for mist, there are several things to look for:

- Observe the mist. If it disappears during inspiration, the oxygen flow to the system is inadequate.

- Some patients may have bronchospasm due to irritation from the aerosol. In this case, a heated, nonaerosol humidification system can be substituted.

- Check the tubing frequently for water collection. Excess water in the tubing can obstruct gas flow.

FIGURE 8-18 T-piece and medication nebulizer.

that the patient can inhale. This is used to administer bronchodilators either preoperatively or postoperatively.

SUCTION

In the OR, suction is used to clear blood, mucus and other secretions from the patient's airway or the surgical site (see Fig. 8-19). Suction also can be used to remove smoke plume from the surgical field. There should always be at least two suction devices available: one for the surgical field and one to help with airway maintenance.

Suction systems consist of several parts. A suction tip or catheter is attached to sterile tubing. The tubing is attached to a vacuum source that is attached to a collection device for the secretions. When activated, the system uses vacuum power to suck the secretions up through the tip/tubing and into the collection device. The vacuum unit can be fixed (e.g., wall suction) or portable. The collection device can be disposable (e.g., rigid plastic container), reusable (e.g., Neptune) or have a disposable liner (e.g., suction carousel).

Suction devices have regulators at the vacuum source so that the strength of the vacuum power can be adjusted. The suction power is expressed in millimeters of mercury (mm Hg). The maximum suction strength depends on the unit, generally varying from −550 mm Hg to −700 mm Hg. The amount of suction used depends on what it is being used for. For wound suction, it is generally set in the high medium range; for suctioning airway secretions, it is generally in the high range (airway secretions are thicker and therefore require a higher vacuum setting).

There are several types of suction tips. The two most commonly used to maintain the airway are the Yankauer (tonsil) and the flexible suction catheter (see Fig. 8-20). The Yankauer or tonsil suction is a long, semirigid tip that is curved toward the end to allow for suctioning the back of the throat. It has a rounded tip with several holes and can suction large amounts of secretions. This suction tip is used to suction the mouth and pharynx. It is available in a reusable (metal) or disposable (plastic) models.

The soft suction catheter is a flexible tube with holes at the end. It has a thumb control at the proximal end that you occlude with your thumb when you want to apply suction (see Fig. 8-21). This suction tip is used to suction the nasopharynx, the oropharynx or inside the ETT. To accommodate suctioning varying sizes of ETTs and patients, the flexible suction catheter is available in sizes 5 Fr to 24 Fr.

ANESTHESIA MACHINERY

Walk into any OR and look toward the head of the bed. What do you see? Usually the answer is the anesthesia machine and a variety of other machines used by anesthesia personnel to provide patient care. This section provides a brief description of the commonly used machines and their use and precautions that OR staff need take.

Anesthesia Machine

The largest and most noticeable machine at the head of the OR bed is the anesthesia machine (see Fig. 8-22), which is needed to administer general anesthesia. It delivers anesthetic gases, air, oxygen and volatile anesthetics to the patient and allows the anesthesia care provider continuously to monitor the patient's vital signs.

There are many different models of anesthesia machine, but most can be divided into its two parts: the anesthetic delivery system and the monitoring system. The monitors usually are positioned on the top of the machine. They allow the anesthesia care provider continuously to monitor the patient's cardiac rhythm (electrocardiogram [ECG]), blood pressure, pulse, end tidal carbon dioxide (end tidal CO_2) and oxygen saturation. In most cases, the monitoring system is configured to allow blood pressure monitoring through the use of a cuff (noninvasive) or an arterial line (invasive).

The anesthetic delivery portion of the machine delivers air, oxygen and nitrous oxide to the patient (either from tanks or wall outlets) and converts the volatile anesthetics to gas vapors that can the patient can breathe. Once general anesthetics have been administered to the patient, this machine allows for manual or mechanical ventilation.

The anesthetic gases are delivered to the patient through a series of hoses that are configured to create a circular flow. This is known as a *circuit*. There are three types of circuit configurations: *open (semiopen), closed* and *semiclosed.*

As the name implies, the *open* system allows atmospheric gases to enter the system; it is "open" to the outside atmosphere. In this system, almost all of the exhaled gases are vented out of the system. All of the gases are vented out of the system instead of being rebreathed, which means that it can be more expensive (increased amount of anesthetic used). This system is used mostly for pediatric patients.

In contrast to the open system, in a *closed* system the patient rebreathes exhaled anesthetic. The exhaled anesthetic is captured and recycled through the circuit. This system uses less anesthetic gases, which means that it can be less expensive to use, and it helps to maintain respiratory humidity and core body temperature.

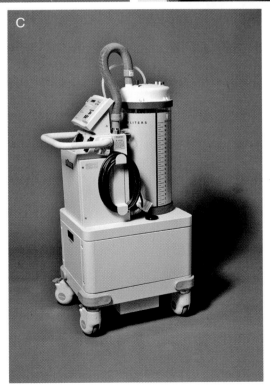

FIGURE 8-19 A) Suction carousel. B) Rigid canister. C) Neptune machine.

In a *semiclosed* system, some anesthetic gases are allowed to escape while some are recycled through the system. In both the open and semiclosed systems, a gas salvaging system is used to capture the exhaled gases. To prevent the patient from rebreathing his or her own carbon dioxide, a soda lime reservoir is part of the circuit (see Fig. 8-23). The soda lime absorbs the carbon dioxide to prevent it from re-entry into the circuit.

FIGURE 8–20 Yankauer suction tips.

FIGURE 8–21 Small and large suction catheters.

FIGURE 8–22 Anesthesia machine.

Another part of the anesthesia machine is the vaporizer (see Fig. 8-24). The vaporizer converts volatile liquid anesthetics such as Desflurane, Sevoflurane and Isoflurane to a gaseous state so they can be inhaled by the patient through the circuit. Each liquid anesthetic has different characteristics; therefore, the machine contains a separate vaporizer for each.

The last part of the machine controls the patient's ventilation. The anesthesia care provider can deliver gases and control the patient's ventilatory rate and volume either manually (by squeezing the bag) or automatically (by switching on the ventilator) (see Fig. 8-25).

Bair Hugger

Intraoperative *hypothermia* (lower than normal body temperature) can lead to a multitude of complications: increased risk of surgical site infection, coagulation problems, increased risk of morbid cardiac events and delayed drug absorption. To help combat intraoperative hypothermia, devices exist that blow forced hot air into a special blanket that is used to continuously warm the patient. The Bair Hugger is one such device (see Fig. 8-26). The temperature can be adjusted to low, medium or high (depending on the patient, length of surgery,

FIGURE 8–23 Soda lime canister.

Cleaning the Anesthesia Machine Between Patients

Decontamination and cleaning of the anesthesia machine between patients may be the responsibility of an anesthesia tech, an anesthesia care provider or the OR staff, depending on the institution. Institutional policies for cleaning and decontamination may vary (be sure to check your institution's policies), but there are some general rules:

- Follow standard precautions when handling any contaminated equipment or supplies.

- Change all equipment that comes in contact with the patient (single-use items such as masks, hoses, ventilation bag, ECG leads) or decontaminate it (blood pressure cuffs, nondisposable pulse oximeter probes, ECG lead wires).

- Change soda lime canisters between patients or when they are used up (the soda lime granules turn purple when they are used; too much purple is an indication that they need to be changed). This is dependent on institutional policy.

- Remove used laryngoscope blades from the room and clean or sterilize them according to your institution's policies.

- Check all hoses to make sure they are connected and snug, not loose.

FIGURE 8–25 Ventilator.

FIGURE 8–24 Vaporizer.

Bair Hugger

- Bair Hugger devices should be used only with the special blanket attached. The unattached hose should NEVER be placed next to the patient's skin or under the regular blankets. Patient *skin burns* have occurred when the hose was used without the blanket!

- Bair Hugger hoses should not be used to warm the sheets prior to the patient's arrival in the OR; heating the sheets could cause a burn or fire. The air from the hose also causes the sheets to flap around and increases the amount air current, which spreads contamination in the OR.

FIGURE 8–26 Bair Hugger.

type of procedure and temperature of the OR). Blankets designed for upper body use and lower body use are available to warm the body area not involved in the surgical procedure.

Blanketrol

The Blanketrol is a device that circulates heated or cooled water through coils in a special blanket, allowing for control of patient body temperature (see Fig. 8-27). The machine can be operated in one of three modes: *automatic* (controls patient temperature), *manual* (controls water temperature) and *monitor* (monitors the patient's temperature through use of a probe). The Blanketrol can be used in warming mode to help prevent intraoperative hypothermia or in cooling mode to help decrease patient body temperature (e.g., in patients with high fevers). Blankets are available for single patient use (e.g., isolation cases) or in reusable styles (made of urethane).

Bispectral Index Monitor

The Bispectral Index (BIS) monitor allows the anesthesia care provider to monitor the patient's level of consciousness under general anesthesia (see Fig. 8-28). The machine takes electroencephalogram (EEG) data from the patient's brain and processes it to come up with a single number that corresponds to the patient's depth of anesthesia. The use of this device may reduce the incidence of patient awareness during anesthesia, and it may reduce the amount of drug needed to ensure amnesia thus leading to faster wake-up times. Numeric values of 40 to 60 have

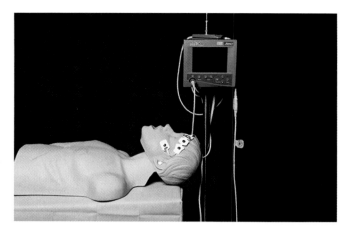

FIGURE 8-28 BIS machine and sensor strip on manikin.

been recommended for ensuring adequate levels of general anesthesia (and patient amnesia).

The monitor is attached to the patient by use of a special sensor strip attached to the patient's forehead. The sensor strip is them attached to a cord coming from the machine.

Syringe Infusion Pump

The model pictured in Figure 8-29 is made by Baxter and called an InfusOR pump. This device is designed so that the anesthesia care provider inserts a syringe of medication (e.g., propofol) and it is infused into the patient's IV at a set rate.

FIGURE 8-27 Blanketrol with blanket.

FIGURE 8-29 Baxter syringe infusion pump.

FIGURE 8-30 Abbott pump.

Infusion rates can be adjusted using dials on the face of the machine. A library of SMART LABELS is available for various commonly used medications. The SMART LABELS are magnetically coded and drug specific. The provider changes the SMART LABEL when he or she inserts a syringe of new medication into the machine. The dosages are already figured on the label thus saving calculation time and decreasing chance of calculation errors.

Patient-Controlled Anesthesia/Epidural Pump

There are several companies that make patient-controlled anesthesia/epidural pumps. The one pictured in Figure 8-30 is made by Abbott. These pumps are programmable, allowing the care provider to set the machine to deliver a pre-set amount of medication to the patient at given intervals. These pumps can be used to deliver medication through an epidural catheter or an IV line. The pump can be programmed to deliver the medication continuously, intermittently (by having the patient push a button) or both. These pumps require special tubing.

Fluid Warmer

There are several fluid/blood warmers on the market. The one pictured in Figure 8-31 is the Hotline warmer. This model uses a warm water bath to heat IV solutions or blood prior to infusion into the patient. Fluids are warmed to between 95°F and 105°F. The fluid is warmed and ready to use in about 4 minutes. Special tubing is required for use with this machine.

Defibrillator

There are many defibrillators on the market. The Zoll model is shown in Figure 8-32. The purpose of a defibrillator is to allow for monitoring, defibrillating, cardioversion or pacing during an untoward cardiac event. Many models use pads for "hands-off" delivery of electricity. The defibrillator pictured allows for use of pads or "paddles" (hands-on). Paddles cannot be used for pacing; therefore, most practitioners prefer to apply the pads because they can be used for any mode.

The electricity delivered to the heart can be either a monophasic or biphasic configuration. Biphasic technology is

FIGURE 8-31 Hotline warmer.

the newer technology. A biphasic defibrillator requires a lower setting of electricity 200 joules maximum, whereas a monophasic defibrillator requires a setting of 360 joules maximum. Make sure you know which type (monophasic or biphasic) of defibrillator your department has, recommended settings, how to operate it safely and how to attach the pads, paddles and internal paddles.

The pads and paddles are for external defibrillation, cardioversion and pacing. The internal paddles require far less energy (10 to 40 joules for an adult) and are applied directly to the heart. They can be only be used if the chest cavity is opened up (e.g., thoracic surgeries, open heart procedures).

Pads, paddles and internal paddles are available in adult and pediatric sizes.

WATCH OUT!	Defibrillators

- Defibrillators should only be used by personnel who know how to operate the machine properly. Injury to the patient or other personnel can occur if used improperly.

- Before pushing the "shock" button to discharge the electrical shock, give a verbal cue (e.g., "I'm clear, you're clear, everyone is clear") and LOOK to make sure no one is touching the patient or the stretcher or bed.

FIGURE 8–32 A) Defibrillator. B) Pads (adult and pediatric).

Transesophageal Echocardiography Scope

The transesophageal echocardiography (TEE) is a fiberoptic scope with an ultrasound transducer connected to the distal end (see Fig. 8-33). The scope and transducer are threaded through the patient's mouth and into the esophagus. The esophagus sits directly behind the heart; therefore, the ultrasound beam has less obstructions to travel through than a standard external ultrasound in which the transducer is placed on the outside of the chest and the beam has to travel through skin, tissue, muscles and ribs. The TEE gives a much clearer picture of the heart. Most modern TEE machines have features that allow for color Doppler imaging of blood flow through the cardiac valves. These types of images are most often done in patients undergoing cardiac surgery, but they could be done for any patient with suspected cardiac disease (especially valve, atrial or ventricular abnormalities). In the OR setting, TEE should be performed by anesthesia providers who are familiar with its use and interpretation.

Fiberoptic Bronchoscopes

Fiberoptic bronchoscopes are used for direct visualization of the respiratory tract and lungs (see Fig. 8-34). These scopes are most often used in the OR for placement of an ETT into a patient who is difficult to intubate using a conventional laryngoscope. They can also be used to place a "double" ETT in a patient who is undergoing lung surgery. Bronchoscopes are available in various sizes including adult and pediatric.

FIGURE 8–33 TEE scope and machine.

FIGURE 8–34 Bronchoscope.

OTHER EQUIPMENT

In this section are pictures and brief descriptions of some of the other equipment that anesthesia care providers use when providing patient care in the OR.

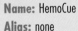

Name: HemoCue

Alias: none

Use: allows bedside testing of the patient's hemoglobin level

Features: quick, accurate test; allows for easy testing intraoperatively

Additional Information: should be used only by those who have been trained in its proper use; test strips should be checked periodically for outdating

Name: Glucometer

Alias: glucose testing machine

Use: allows bedside testing of the patient's blood sugar level

Features: quick, accurate test; allows for easy testing intraoperatively

Additional Information: should be used only by those who have been trained in its proper use; test strips should be checked periodically for outdating

Name: Propaq

Alias: transport monitor

Use: monitors cardiac rhythm and vital signs during transport

Features: small, compact size makes for easy portability

Additional Information: able to monitor ECG, oxygen saturation, pulse and blood pressure

Name: temperature monitoring disc

Alias: none

Use: is placed on patient's forehead to monitor skin surface temperature during surgery

Features: peel-off backing allows for adhesion to the patient's skin

Additional Information: single patient use

Name: Braslow tape

Alias: none

Use: estimates weight of pediatric patients for medication dosage calculation

Features: color-coded by weight; has common emergency medication calculations written on it by weight; tells what size of tubes and so on to use according to estimated weight; weight is estimated according to child's height: lay the marked end of the tape at the child's head and where the bottom of his or her feet fall is the estimated weight

Additional Information: laminated for easy cleaning between patients; has calculations up to 34 kg

Name: esophageal stethoscope

Alias: none

Use: monitors heart and breath sounds during surgery

Features: is hooked up to a fitted earpiece to allow for the anesthesia care provider to monitor heart/breath sounds while listening to other OR sounds/communication

Additional Information: inserted by anesthesia care provider after patient is asleep and intubated

Name: oxygen saturation probe

Alias: none

Use: measures the oxygen saturation present in the patient's hemoglobin

Features: noninvasive; probe clips onto finger or toe

Additional Information: available with reusable or disposable probes

Name: cerebral oxygen monitor

Alias: none

Use: measures the oxygen level in the brain; used during procedures such as carotid endarterectomy to monitor cerebral blood flow

Features: disposable pads can be placed on either (or both) side of the patient's forehead for monitoring

Additional Information: none

Name: skin temperature sensor

Alias: none

Use: enables intraoperative skin temperature monitoring

Features: adhesive side has a tiny probe embedded that is touching the skin to monitor the skin temperature

Additional Information: plug end is attached to the temperature monitor

Name: Tubex holder

Alias: none

Use: holds medication to allow for injection

Features: accepts standard Tubex medication cartridges

Additional Information: reusable

Name: ECG leads

Alias: monitor electrodes

Use: are placed on the chest to allow for attachment of ECG monitoring electrodes

Features: self-adhesive

Additional Information: available in adult and pediatric sizes; single use only

Name: Bullard laryngoscope

Alias: none

Use: aids in visualizing the airway when there is an inability to align the axes of the airway, such as in patients with upper body burns, unstable cervical fractures, anterior larynx or temporomandibular joint immobility

Features: rigid; needs a fiberoptic light source; can be used in a patient whose mouth opening is as little as 6 mm; can be used to aid in nasal and oral intubations

Additional Information: available in pediatric and adult sizes

BLOCK NEEDLES AND SUPPLIES

Name: Sprotte spinal needle

Alias: none

Use: creates a pathway for the introduction of regional anesthetics into the spinal canal for spinal analgesia/anesthesia; can be used to inject medication into deep or hard to reach areas (e.g., cervix)

Features: 3.5 to 5 inches long; pencil tip point; designed for atraumatic dural puncture; "noncutting point"

Additional Information: available in 22-gauge to 29-gauge sizes; available with or without an introducer

Name: Quincke spinal needle

Alias: none

Use: creates a pathway for the introduction of regional anesthetics into the spinal canal for spinal analgesia/anesthesia; can be used to inject medication into deep or hard to reach areas (e.g., cervix)

Features: 90-mm long; sharp, cutting point

Additional Information: available in 18-gauge to 29-gauge sizes; available with or without an introducer

Name: Whitacre spinal needle

Alias: none

Use: creates a pathway for the introduction of regional anesthetics into the spinal canal for spinal analgesia/anesthesia; can be used to inject medication into deep or hard to reach areas (e.g., cervix)

Features: pencil point tip; 3.5- to 5.5-inches long

Additional Information: available in 18-gauge to 27-gauge sizes; available in regular or high-flow style

Name: regional block needle

Alias: security bead needle

Use: administers medication for regional nerve blocks

Features: 1.5-inch long security bead on the shaft of the needle to prevent overinsertion

Additional Information: available in 20- and 22-gauge sizes

Name: spinal block kit

Alias: none

Use: used to insert needle for administration of spinal anesthesia

Features: contains all needed supplies and equipment to administer spinal anesthesia

Additional Information: practitioner may choose to add additional supplies per personal preference; inside of the kit is considered sterile

Name: epidural kit

Alias: none

Use: used to insert epidural catheter for administration of epidural anesthesia

Features: contains all needed supplies and equipment to administer epidural anesthesia

Additional Information: practitioner may choose to add additional supplies per personal preference; inside of the kit is considered sterile

Name: Touchy epidural needle

Alias: none

Use: inserts into the epidural space to allow passage of an epidural catheter

Features: finger control (wings)

Additional Information: available in 16-gauge to 22-gauge sizes, 40-mm (pediatric) to 160-mm lengths

Name: epidural catheter

Alias: none

Use: used to administer medication into the epidural space for regional anesthesia or analgesia

Features: can stay in the patient's back for several days postoperatively to provide analgesic medication

Additional Information: comes in a variety of sizes and lengths

Name: Stimuplex

Alias: nerve stimulator

Use: stimulates nerves; used for insertion of regional nerve blocks

Features: output control can be adjusted for higher or lower stimulation

Additional Information: use with disposable Stimuplex needle

Name: Stimuplex needle

Alias: nerve block needle

Use: inserts into the nerve plexus to allow for injection of regional anesthetic

Features: attaches to Stimuplex machine; single patient use

Additional Information: needs to be irrigated prior to insertion into patient; available in 4- and 1.5-inch lengths

IV SUPPLIES AND SOLUTIONS

Name: central venous pressure monitoring kit

Alias: CVP line kit

Use: used to monitor the patient's fluid status by monitoring the pressure in the vena cava and right atrium

Features: kit comes with everything needed to insert the line

Additional Information: none

Name: IV catheters

Alias: IV needles

Use: starts an IV infusion on a patient

Features: safety needle; once the catheter is in place, the white button is pushed and the needle retracts into the plastic sheath

Additional Information: come in a variety of gauges (16, 18, 20, 22 and 24 gauge are the most common sizes); the larger the gauge number, the small the catheter diameter (e.g., a size 16 catheter has a much larger diameter than a size 24)

Name: tourniquet

Alias: none

Use: starts IV infusions; may be used in a dire emergency to control bleeding from limbs

Features: some have Velcro closures; most are latex-free

Additional Information: comes in a variety of sizes and styles

Name: Walrus tubing

Alias: anesthesia IV tubing

Use: connects IV solution to IV catheter

Features: multiple stopcocks for injection of medications during induction and intraoperatively

Additional Information: latex-free

Name: extension set

Alias: none

Use: extends the length of IV tubing; attach to IV catheter to extend saline lock site

Features: comes in a variety of lengths

Additional Information: single use

Name: sodium chloride 0.9%

Alias: normal saline

Use: provides fluid replacement or volume expansion

Features: isotonic solution; does not contain potassium

Additional Information: available in several sizes of bags (50 mL, 100 mL, 250 mL, 500 mL, 1000 mL)

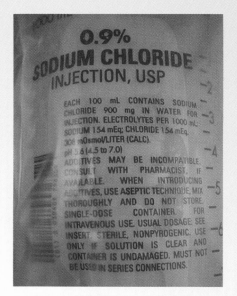

Name: Lactated Ringer's

Alias: LR

Use: provides fluid replacement or volume expansion

Features: electrolyte solution; contains sodium, potassium, calcium and chloride

Additional Information: available in several sizes of bags (250 mL, 500 mL, 1000 mL)

Name: butterfly infusion set

Alias: none

Use: used to draw blood; instill IV solutions or medication

Features: uses a metal needle rather than a plastic catheter that stays in the patient's vein; needle tends to be shorter than an IV catheter, sometimes making it easier to dislodge

Additional Information: available in a variety of gauges (19, 21, 23 and 25 gauge are the most common)

Name: three-way stopcock

Alias: none

Use: allows more than one medication or fluid to be administered in rapid succession, such as a medication that needs to be followed with a saline flush

Features: lever turns to allow opening and closing of each port

Additional Information: available in plastic (disposable) or metal (resterilizable)

Name: alcohol wipe

Alias: prep pad

Use: cleans the skin prior to IV insertion; cleans the port prior to injection of medication

Features: comes ready to use; contains isopropyl alcohol

Additional Information: none

Name: arterial line needles

Alias: none

Use: inserted into an artery, it allows access for monitoring, blood drawing or administration of fluids and medications

Features: has slider to allow for easier insertion once the artery is cannulated

Additional Information: available in short or long sizes

Name: dextrose 5%

Alias: D5W

Use: acts as a glucose and fluid replacement

Features: contains glucose for sugar replacement

Additional Information: dextrose provides calories to patient

Name: IV pressure bag

Alias: none

Use: exerts pressure on IV solution bags to increase flow rate

Features: has a pressure gauge to measure pressure being exerted

Additional Information: available in several styles

Name: T connector

Alias: none

Use: connects IV catheter to adapter to create a saline or heparin lock

Features: the "T" plugs into the IV catheter and an adapter goes on the other end; has a slide clamp to allow it to be occluded when not in use

Additional Information: none

Name: microdrip tubing

Alias: none

Use: administers small amounts of IV solution or medication to a patient; used when patient fluid intake needs to be limited or on pediatric patients

Features: small drip size: 60 drops equals 1 mL

Additional Information: none

Name: secondary IV tubing

Alias: piggyback tubing

Use: piggyback medication drips into main IV line

Features: comes with plastic hanger for main IV bag and blunt needle to use to insert it into the main IV line

Additional Information: main IV should be hung below the piggyback IV bag using the plastic hanger

Name: burette

Alias: none

Use: measures and administers small amounts of IV medication or fluid; used most commonly with pediatric patients; microdrip administration system

Features: chamber allows for the measuring out and administration of restricted amounts of fluid; IV bag can be shut off after the fluid is measured into the chamber so that only the fluid in the chamber is given

Additional Information: 150-mL capacity chamber

Name: blood administration set

Alias: Y-tubing

Use: used to administer blood

Features: double spikes allow blood bag and saline IV bag to be hung together; filter built into the tubing

Additional Information: none

Name: arterial line set up

Alias: none

Use: allows for pressure measurements directly from the artery as well as blood drawing

Features: IV bag is heparinized saline to keep the line from clotting off; can be set up for one, two or three transducers (to allow for central venous pressure [CVP] monitoring as well)

Additional Information: set up may vary by institution or equipment

---

| WATCH OUT! | Needle Safety |

When handling injectable, IV or regional block needles, there are several safety precautions that should be taken to minimize the risk of needle-stick injury to oneself or others.

- Use IV or injectable needles that have safety sheaths on them whenever possible. Activate the safety sheath as soon as you are finished with the needle.

- Use a "needle-less" system to inject medications into IV tubing whenever available. If your institution does not have a needle-less IV tubing system, use blunt needles, if available, to inject medication into the ports.

- When possible, load needles onto syringes just prior to use. Do not leave syringes and needles lying around unattended.

- Know where your needles are at all times. Keep track of where you or the person you are assisting is placing the sharps.

- Place all used needles in a puncture-proof disposal container.

- Never recap used needles with your hands. If you must recap a needle, use the "scoop" method or a recapping device.

- Never use your hands to bend or break needles.

MEDICATIONS

Name: adenosine

Alias: Adenocard

Medication Class: antiarrhythmic

Use: treats narrow, complex tachycardias

Features: each vial contains 6 mg; very short half-life, must be given via IV push over 1 to 2 seconds and followed by a 20-cc saline bolus

Additional Information: initial dose is 6 mg; up to two more doses of 12 mg each may be given if needed

Name: albumin

Alias: albumin 5%; albumin 25%

Medication Class: volume expander

Use: restores plasma volume during cardiac bypass procedures or during treatment of burns or shock

Features: acts by expanding the volume of circulating blood and maintaining cardiac output

Additional Information: 5% albumin is used to treat shock; 5% albumin is generally used initially and 25% may be used after 24 hours

Name: albuterol

Alias: Proventil, Ventolin, Volmax

Medication Class: bronchodilator

Use: prevents/treats wheezing, bronchospasm

Features: medication can be used with the inhaler or can be squirted down the ETT.

Additional Information: usual dose is one to two puffs

Name: alfentanil hydrochloride

Alias: Alfenta; Rapifen

Medication Class: opioid; narcotic analgesic

Use: relieves pain (analgesic)

Features: makes the patient drowsy; alters pain perception and response; can cause respiratory depression

Additional Information: usual dose depends on length of anesthesia required

Name: Alupent

Alias: metaproterenol

Medication Class: bronchodilator

Use: prevents/treats wheezing, bronchospasm

Features: can be given PO or via inhaler; inhaler can be squirted down the ETT

Additional Information: usual dosage is two to three puffs every 3 to 4 hours (not to exceed 12 puffs/day); PO dosage 10 mg to 20 mg every 6 to 8 hours

Name: amiodarone

Alias: Cordarone

Medication Class: antiarrhythmic

Use: treats wide complex tachycardias; also may be used to treat cardiac arrest

Features: must be diluted in D5W prior to infusion

Additional Information: usual dose for cardiac arrest is 300 mg given IV via push; usual dose for treatment of tachycardia is 150 mg (diluted in 100 cc of D5W) given via IV drip

Name: ampicillin

Alias: Omnipen; Polycillin

Medication Class: broad-spectrum antibiotic

Use: helps prevent postoperative infection

Features: can be given PO, IM or IV; reconstituted and given preoperatively via IV piggyback; cannot be used for patients with penicillin allergies

Additional Information: usual IV dose is 1 g to 2 g

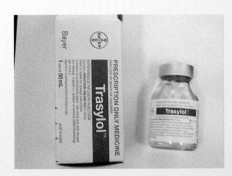

Name: aprotinin

Alias: Trasylol

Medication Class: antifibrinolytic

Use: decreases bleeding complications associated with cardiac bypass surgery

Features: should be administered via IV through a central line; no other medication should be given through this line

Additional Information: dosing includes a 1-mL test dose, a 1 million– to 2 million–unit IV dose and a 1 million– to 2 million–unit dose added to the recirculating priming fluid in the bypass pump, followed with a continuous infusion

Name: artificial tears

Alias: Akwa Tears

Medication Class: eye lubricant

Use: prevent corneal drying during anesthesia

Features: come in ointment form; some brands of artificial tears come as drops

Additional Information: apply to each eye as needed during general anesthesia

Name: atropine

Alias: none

Medication Class: anticholinergic; antiarrhythmic

Use: increases heart rate in bradycardic arrhythmias; can be used preoperatively to decrease secretions

Features: each bristojet contains 1 mg; also comes in vials; can cause dryness of mouth/mucous membranes

Additional Information: dose is 0.5 to 1.0 mg; given via IV push for arrhythmias; preoperative dosage is 0.4 mg to 0.6 mg (adult) and 0.1 mg to 0.4 mg (pediatric)

Name: Bicitra

Alias: citra pH

Medication Class: antacid

Use: reduces gastric pH

Features: given PO

Additional Information: usual dose is 15 to 30 cc (may be diluted with water on a 50:50 mixture)

Name: buprenorphine

Alias: Buprenex

Medication Class: opioid; narcotic analgesic

Use: relieves pain (analgesic)

Features: may be given IM or IV; can cause drowsiness in patients

Additional Information: usual dose is 0.3 mg to 0.6 mg every 6 hours as needed (reduce dosage for elderly patients)

Name: caffeine

Alias: none

Medication Class:

Use: treats migraine headaches; prevents caffeine-induced headaches

Features: given via IV drip-mix with D5W or normal saline

Additional Information: none

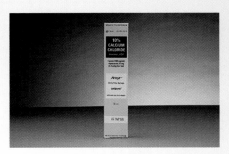

Name: calcium chloride 10%

Alias: none

Medication Class: electrolyte replacement

Use: prevents and treats hypocalcemia

Features: each bristojet contains 1 g

Additional Information: usual dose is 500 mg to 1 g based on serum calcium levels

Name: cefazolin

Alias: Ancef; Kefzol

Medication Class: antibiotic (cephalosporin)

Use: helps prevent postoperative infection

Features: diluted and given via IV piggyback or push; can be given preoperatively, intraoperatively or postoperatively

Additional Information: usual dose is 1 to 2 g; use with caution in patients with penicillin allergies

Name: cefotetan

Alias: Cefotan

Medication Class: second-generation cephalosporin antibiotic

Use: helps prevent postoperative infection

Features: diluted and given via IV piggyback or push; can be given preoperatively, intraoperatively or postoperatively

Additional Information: usual dose is 500 mg to 1 g

Name: clindamycin

Alias: Cleocin

Medication Class: antibiotic

Use: helps prevent postoperative infection

Features: diluted in NS or D5W and given via IV infusion

Additional Information: usual dose is 400 mg to 600 mg infusion

Name: clonidine

Alias: Catapres

Medication Class: antihypertensive; analgesic

Use: treats hypertension; treats vascular headaches

Features: can be given PO, transdermally or via continuous epidural infusion

Additional Information: usual PO dose is 0.2 to 0.8 mg/day in divided doses; usual epidural dose is 30 µg/hour (adult)

Name: chloroprocaine

Alias: Nesacaine

Medication Class: local anesthetic

Use: used as epidural anesthesia, peripheral nerve block, caudal anesthesia, infiltration of site

Features: duration 0.5 to 1 hour

Additional Information: can cause cardiac arrhythmias and hypotension; needs continuous monitoring throughout the procedure

Name: clopidogrel

Alias: Plavix

Medication Class: platelet inhibitor

Use: reduces the risk of stroke in high-risk patients

Features: do not give to patients with active bleeding; puts patients at risk for increased bleeding; given PO

Additional Information: usual dose is 75 mg/day

Name: cocaine

Alias: none

Medication Class: topical anesthetic

Use: used as topical anesthesia in nasal procedures; is a vasoconstrictor so it reduces nasal bleeding

Features: can be swabbed on the nasal mucosa or cocaine-soaked cottonoids can be inserted into the nares

Additional Information: for topical use only

Name: dantrolene

Alias: Dantrium

Medication Class: skeletal muscle relaxant

Use: treats malignant hyperthermia

Features: comes in a powder form, must be diluted with sterile water

Additional Information: loading dose is 2.5 mg/kg mixed with injectable sterile water; using teams of two people to mix it makes for easier and faster mixing

---

Name: Demerol

Alias: meperidine

Medication Class: opioid; narcotic analgesic

Use: relieves pain (analgesic)

Features: can be given IV or IM; may make patient nauseated; makes patient drowsy

Additional Information: dosages range from 25 mg to 100 mg IM or 25 to 50 mg IV

Name: dexamethasone

Alias: Decadron; Hexadrol; Mymethasone

Medication Class: corticosteroid (anti-inflammatory)

Use: prevents/reduces inflammation and edema

Features: can be given PO, IM or IV; may be used topically during surgery (e.g., spine surgery); can be injected directly into a joint

Additional Information: dose varies depending on route and use

Name: desflurane

Alias: Suprane

Medication Class: inhalation anesthetic

Use: induces and maintains anesthesia

Features: more rapid onset and recovery than some other gases; strong odor

Additional Information: requires the use of a heated vaporizer for administration

Name: Dextrose 50%

Alias: none

Medication Class: carbohydrate

Use: increases blood sugar in severe hypoglycemia

Features: each bristojet contains 25 g of dextrose

Additional Information: average adult dose is 25 to 50 g IV push

Name: Diamox

Alias: acetazolamide

Medication Class: diuretic

Use: reduces edema associated with glaucoma or congestive heart failure (CHF)

Features: can be given PO, IM or IV

Additional Information: dosage depends on use

Name: Dilaudid

Alias: hydromorphone

Medication Class: opioid; narcotic analgesic

Use: pain reliever (analgesic)

Features: makes patient drowsy; can cause respiratory depression; can be given PO, IM, IV or rectally

Additional Information: usual IM or IV dose is 2 mg to 4 mg every 4 to 6 hours

Name: diphenhydramine

Alias: Benadryl

Medication Class: antihistamine

Use: treats allergic reactions, motion sickness, insomnia and cough

Features: can be given PO, IM, IV; may cause drowsiness

Additional Information: common ingredient in most over-the-counter allergy medications

Name: Diprivan
Alias: propofol
Medication Class: general anesthetic
Use: inducts or maintains anesthesia; sedates patients on ventilators
Features: given IV; do not mix with other agents in the same syringe
Additional Information: to be used only by personnel trained in anesthesia administration

Name: dobutamine
Alias: Dobutrex
Medication Class: catecholamine
Use: can be used during cardiac surgery; used to treat shock or refractory heart failure
Features: increases cardiac contractility and coronary blood flow; increases heart rate
Additional Information: given IV infusion at a rate of 2.5 to 10 µg/kg/min

Name: dopamine
Alias: Intropin
Medication Class: catecholamine
Use: treats shock and hypotension
Features: comes as a premixed drip
Additional Information: dose is 2 to 5 µg/kg/min (not to exceed 50 µg/kg/min); given as an IV drip; careful monitoring of blood pressure is required

Name: droperidol
Alias: Inapsine
Medication Class: Neuroleptic
Use: antiemetic; used as premedication for surgery; induces and maintains general anesthesia
Features: produces sedation and sleep; can be given IM or IV
Additional Information: dose depends on intended use

Name: edrophonium

Alias: Reversol; Tensilon

Medication Class: anticholinesterase

Use: reverses nondepolarizing neuromuscular blockers

Features: given via IV push

Additional Information: usual dose is 10 mg administered over 30 to 45 seconds; often given concurrently with atropine or Robinul (if given alone, it can cause bradycardia)

Name: ephedrine

Alias: ephedrine sulfate

Medication Class: bronchodilator; adrenergic

Use: treats hypotension and shock; increases perfusion; bronchodilator

Features: causes increased heart rate and cardiac contractility; vasoconstricts blood vessels; given IM, SC or IV to treat shock; may also be given PO if used as a bronchodilator

Additional Information: usual adult dose to treat hypotension is 10 to 25 mg IV (not to exceed 150 mg/day); usual pediatric dose is 3 mg/kg/day

---

Name: epinephrine 1:1000

Alias: adrenaline

Medication Class: bronchodilator; catecholamine

Use: counteracts allergic reactions; treats bronchospasm and asthma

Features: is 10 times stronger than the cardiac epinephrine: DO NOT confuse the two medications; each ampule contains 1 mL; can be given IM, SC, or IV

Additional Information: dose is 0.1 to 0.5 cc SC

Name: epinephrine 1:10,000

Alias: adrenaline

Medication Class: bronchodilator; catecholamine

Use: used during cardiac arrest

Features: each bristojet equals 1 mg

Additional Information: dose is 1 mg every 3 to 5 minutes during cardiac arrest; given via IV push

Name: esmolol

Alias: Brevibloc

Medication Class: antiarrhythmic

Use: treats hypertension and tachycardia

Features: slows heart rate, decreases myocardial oxygen consumption; should not be used in patients with second- or third-degree heart block, CHF or cardiogenic shock

Additional Information: adult loading dose is 500 µg/kg over 1 minute; usual pediatric dose is 50 µg/kg/min

---

Name: etidocaine HCl

Alias: Duranest

Medication Class: local anesthetic

Use: used for peripheral nerve block, spinal anesthesia, caudal anesthesia

Features: duration 3 to 6 hours; available in 1% and 1.5%

Additional Information: dose varies with route of anesthesia; vital signs and ECG need to be monitored during treatment

---

Name: etomidate

Alias: Amidate

Medication Class: general anesthetic

Use: induces general anesthesia

Features: given IV

Additional Information: usual dose is 0.2 to 0.6 mg/kg over 30 to 60 seconds

---

Name: fentanyl citrate

Alias: Sublimaze

Medication Class: opioid; narcotic analgesic

Use: relieves pain (analgesic)

Features: alters pain perception and increases the pain threshold; makes the patient drowsy; 100 µg of fentanyl is the analgesic equivalent of 10 mg of morphine or 75 mg of Demerol

Additional Information: usual dose is 25 µg to 50 µg IV; also available in patch form

Name: furosemide

Alias: Lasix

Medication Class: diuretic

Use: usually used to remove excess fluid from the lungs

Features: comes 10 mg/mL

Additional Information: usual dose is 20 to 80 mg IV push

Name: gentamicin

Alias: none

Medication Class: antibiotic

Use: helps prevent postoperative infection; used frequently in patients undergoing genitourinary procedures

Features: diluted and given via IV piggyback; if the patient is on the medication for several days, he or she should have blood drawn to check medication levels; overdosage can cause ototoxicity and/or nephrotoxicity

Additional Information: usual dose is 60 to 80 mg IV

Name: glycopyrrolate

Alias: Robinul

Medication Class: cholinergic blocker

Use: decreases gastric secretions preoperatively; reverses neuromuscular blockade

Features: may be given PO, IM or IV (route depends on intended use)

Additional Information: usual preoperative dose is 0.002 mg/kg IM; neuromuscular reversal dose is 0.2 mg for each 1 mg of neostigmine (given via IV)

Name: halothane

Alias: Fluothane

Medication Class: inhalation anesthetic

Use: induces and maintains general anesthesia

Features: does not increase heart rate; pleasant odor; causes uterine relaxation and bronchodilation

Additional Information: may cause bradycardia; sensitizes the heart to the arrhythmogenic effects of catecholamines

Name: heparin

Alias: none

Medication Class: anticoagulant

Use: prevents embolus or thrombus formation; treats DVT

Features: available in several concentrations—be sure to read label to know how many units/mL it contains; can be given via IV, SC or IV infusion; during vascular surgery, heparinized saline may be injected directly into the vessels

Additional Information: watch for signs of increased bleeding or hemorrhage; peak IV onset is 5 minutes; dosage depends on use

Name: Hespan

Alias: hetastarch

Medication Class: plasma expander

Use: expands circulatory volume

Features: expands the blood volume one to two times the amount infused

Additional Information: usual dose is 30 to 60 g (500 to 1000 mL); should not exceed 20 mg/kg/hour

Name: hydralazine

Alias: Apresoline, Supres

Medication Class: antihypertensive

Use: treats hypertension

Features: can be given PO, IM or IV

Additional Information: usual IV dose is 20 to 40 mg every 4 to 6 hours

Name: hydrocortisone

Alias: Cortef; Solu-Cortef

Medication Class: corticosteroid

Use: prevents or decreases inflammation

Features: can be given PO, IM or IV; drug can mask signs of infection

Additional Information: usual IM or IV dose is 100 mg to 250 mg

Name: Inderal

Alias: propranolol

Medication Class: antihypertensive; antianginal

Use: treats hypertension, chronic stable angina and migraine prophylaxis

Features: can be given PO or IV; should not be used in patients with second- or third-degree heart block, hypotension, CHF or bradycardia

Additional Information: IV dose is 0.5 mg to 3 mg: give at a rate of 1 mg/min

Name: Indigo Carmine

Alias: none

Medication Class: dye

Use: used to check for unintentional surgical holes in the urinary system

Features: given via IV and excreted by the renal system

Additional Information: none

Name: isoflurane

Alias: Forane

Medication Class: inhalation anesthetic

Use: induces and maintains general anesthesia

Features: rapid induction and recovery

Additional Information: causes profound respiratory depression

Name: isoproterenol

Alias: Isuprel

Medication Class: catecholamine

Use: treats heart block, shock, bronchospasm, asthma

Features: given via IV infusion for treatment of shock or arrhythmias; given sublingual (SL) or inhalation for treatment of asthma or bronchospasm

Additional Information: usual IV infusion dose is 5 μg/min; can cause tissue sloughing if the IV infiltrates; IV infusion is mixed in D5W

Name: ketamine

Alias: Ketalar, Ketanest, Ketaset

Medication Class: general anesthetic; dissociative agent

Use: helps to produce a rapid anesthetic induction

Features: can be given IM or IV

Additional Information: does not provide relaxation (needs to be used with other medications); can produce vivid imagery and hallucinations

Name: Kytril

Alias: granisetron

Medication Class: antiemetic

Use: prevents nausea and vomiting

Features: can be given PO or IV

Additional Information: dilute in NaCl or D5W for IV direct administration

Name: labetalol

Alias: Normodyne

Medication Class: antihypertensive

Use: treats hypertension

Features: can be given PO or IV; should not be used in patients with cardiogenic shock, heart block, bradycardia, CHF or asthma

Additional Information: onset of action is 5 minutes if given IV; usual IV dose is 20 mg given over 2 minutes; may repeat 40 to 80 mg every 10 minutes; do not exceed 300 mg total

Name: levobupivacaine

Alias: Chirocaine

Medication Class: local anesthetic

Use: used as local and regional anesthesia; pain management; continuous epidural infusion

Features: duration of 3 to 6 hours

Additional Information: dose depends on route of anesthesia given; vital signs and ECG need to be monitored during anesthesia

Name: lidocaine

Alias: Xylocaine

Medication Class: local anesthetic

Use: used as local and regional anesthesia

Features: can be given PO (viscous Xylocaine), local injection around the site, IV (e.g., Bair block) or topically (Xylocaine ointment or cream)

Additional Information: comes with and without epinephrine added; red lettering is present on the packaging of bottles that contain epinephrine; usual concentrations are 1%, 2% and 4%

Name: lidocaine (cardiac)

Alias: Xylocaine

Medication Class: antiarrhythmic

Use: controls ventricular arrhythmias

Features: each bristojet contains 100 mg; also comes in vials; must be PRESERVATIVE FREE for cardiac use

Additional Information: dose is 1.0 to 1.5 mg/kg (average dose 75 to 100 mg); may repeat up to two more doses, 5 minutes apart; maximum dose 225 mg; given via IV push

Name: LMD 10%

Alias: low molecular weight dextrose; dextran 40

Medication Class: volume expander

Use: used for plasma volume expansion

Features: given via IV infusion; expands blood volume one to two times the amount infused

Additional Information: usual dose is 500 mL over 15 to 30 minutes

Name: Lovenox

Alias: enoxaparin

Medication Class: anticoagulant

Use: prevents pulmonary embolus and/or deep venous thrombosis in patients undergoing hip or knee replacement surgery or abdominal surgery

Features: given SC for 7 to 10 days postoperatively

Additional Information: should not be given to patients with pork allergies; should not be used in patients with bleeding disorders or history of bleeding problems; usual dose is 30 mg SC twice a day

Name: magnesium sulfate

Alias: none

Medication Class: electrolyte

Use: treats low serum magnesium, torsades de pointes and pre-eclampsia/eclampsia

Features: can be given PO, IM or IV

Additional Information: dosage depends on condition being treated

Name: mannitol

Alias: none

Medication Class: osmotic diuretic

Use: decreases cerebral edema; decreases intraocular pressure; improves renal function for patients in acute renal failure

Features: increases urinary output and sodium excretion; can cause dehydration; needs to be administered with a filter in the IV line

Additional Information: usual IV dose is 1 to 2 g/kg of a 15% or 25% solution over 0.5 hour to 1 hour; Foley catheter should be in place when this medication is being used

Name: Marcaine

Alias: Sensorcaine; bupivacaine

Medication Class: local anesthetic

Use: used as local and regional anesthesia

Features: four times more potent than lidocaine

Additional Information: available with or without epinephrine added—red lettering is present on the packaging of those bottles containing epinephrine; available in various strengths (e.g., 0.25%, 0.5%, 0.75%)

Name: methadone

Alias: Dolophine

Medication Class: opiate analgesic

Use: controls severe pain; opiate withdrawal

Features: can be given PO, SC or IM; may cause drowsiness and respiratory depression

Additional Information: usual adult dose is 2.5 mg to 10 mg every 4 to 12 hours

Name: methylene blue

Alias: none

Medication Class: staining agent; dye

Use: stains surgical site; checks patency of fallopian tubes during tuboplasty

Features: injected into intended site, it creates a blue stain

Additional Information: none

Name: methylprednisolone

Alias: Medrol; Depo-Medrol; Solu-Medrol

Medication Class: corticosteroid

Use: treats severe inflammation, adrenal insufficiency, shock

Features: can be given PO, IM or IV; should not be given to patients younger than 2 years or those with tuberculosis or AIDS

Additional Information: usual dose for treatment of shock is 100 to 250 mg IV every 2 to 6 hours; usual adult dose for treatment of inflammation is 10 to 250 mg IV

Name: metoprolol

Alias: Betaloc, Lopressor, Toprol

Medication Class: antihypertensive; antianginal

Use: treats mild to moderate hypertension; controls angina pectoris; used in the setting of acute myocardial infarction to reduce cardiovascular mortality

Features: can be given PO or IV; should not be used in patients with heart block, cardiogenic shock, bradycardia or bronchial asthma

Additional Information: usual IV dose is 5 mg every 2 minutes for three doses

Name: metronidazole

Alias: Flagyl

Medication Class: anti-infective

Use: treats or prevents infection

Features: can be given PO or IV; has an immediate onset if given IV; may cause vision problems

Additional Information: usual IV dose is 15 mg/kg infused over 1 hour

Name: mivacurium

Alias: Mivacron

Medication Class: nondepolarizing neuromuscular blocker

Use: causes skeletal muscle relaxation; facilitates intubation

Features: given via IV; peak onset is 2 to 3 minutes with reversal in 15 to 30 minutes

Additional Information: usual adult dose is 0.15 mg/kg

Name: morphine sulfate

Alias: morphine

Medication Class: opioid; narcotic analgesic

Use: relieves pain (analgesic)

Features: can be given IV or IM; may make patient nauseated; makes patient drowsy

Additional Information: usual dose is 1 mg to 10 mg IV push

Name: naloxone

Alias: Narcan

Medication Class: narcotic antagonist

Use: acts as a reversal agent for narcotics

Features: may lead to sudden onset of pain (due to reversal of narcotic effect), which may lead to hypertension and tachycardia

Additional Information: usual dose is 0.4 mg to 2.0 mg

Name: Nardil

Alias: phenelzine

Medication Class: monoamine oxidase inhibitor (MAOI), antidepressant

Use: treats depression, migraine headaches

Features: given PO

Additional Information: usual adult dose is 45 to 60 mg/day in divided doses; can cause hypertensive crisis

Name: Neo-Synephrine

Alias: phenylephrine

Medication Class: adrenergic

Use: treats hypotension and shock; maintains blood pressure during spinal anesthesia; decreases bleeding during nasal surgery

Features: causes vasoconstriction; can be given SC, IM, IV or nasal spray

Additional Information: usual adult IV dose to treat hypotension is 0.1 mg to 0.5 mg; may repeat every 10 to 15 minutes as needed

Name: Nimbex

Alias: cisatracurium

Medication Class: nondepolarizing neuromuscular blocker

Use: causes skeletal muscle relaxation; facilitates intubation

Features: given IV; duration of action is 30 to 40 minutes

Additional Information: usual adult dose is 0.15 to 0.2 mg/kg

Name: nitroglycerin

Alias: Nitro-Bid; Nitrol, NitroQuick

Medication Class: antianginal

Use: treats pain associated with angina pectoris; can be used to decrease preload and afterload in CHF; can be used to create controlled hypotension in surgical procedures

Features: causes coronary vessel vasodilation; can be given sublingual (SL), IV, topically (paste) or transdermally (patch)

Additional Information: dosage depends on the form of medication being used; IV infusion comes in glass bottles (medication is absorbed into the polyvinyl of infusion bags); usual adult IV infusion dose is 5 μg/min to start and then increase by 5 μg every 3 to 5 minutes until you reach the desired effect

Name: nitroprusside

Alias: Nitropress

Medication Class: antihypertensive

Use: treats hypertensive crisis; induces controlled hypotension to decrease bleeding during surgery; treats CHF and cardiogenic shock

Features: onset of action is 1 to 2 minutes; given IV infusion; wrap infusion bottle in aluminum foil to protect from light exposure; infuse using an infusion pump

Additional Information: usual adult dose is 0.5 µg to 8 µg/kg/min; dilute medication in 250 to 1000 mL of D5W

Name: nitrous oxide

Alias: none

Medication Class: inhalation anesthetic

Use: used in conjunction with other agents to provide balanced anesthesia

Features: has little effect on heart rate or blood pressure; not potent enough to be used alone for general anesthesia

Additional Information: gas diffuses into closed spaces thus making it contraindicated for some surgeries (e.g., tympanoplasty)

Name: norepinephrine

Alias: Levophed

Medication Class: catecholamine

Use: treats acute hypotension and shock

Features: onset of action is 1 to 2 minutes; causes increased contractility of the heart, peripheral vasoconstriction and improved coronary blood flow

Additional Information: usual adult dose is 8 to 12 µg/min; titrate to desired blood pressure

Name: Nubain

Alias: nalbuphine

Medication Class: opiate analgesic

Use: controls moderate to severe pain; supplements balanced anesthesia

Features: can be given SC, IM or IV; may cause drowsiness or respiratory depression

Additional Information: usual adult dose is 10 to 20 mg every 3 to 6 hours as needed

Name: oxygen

Alias: none

Medication Class: essential gas

Use: provides supplemental oxygen to organs and tissue

Features: can be given via cannula, mask or Ambu bag; flow rate for cannula should be 1 to 3 L; a flow rate of 8 to 10 L is best for a mask; a flow rate of 10 to 15 L is needed for an Ambu bag

Additional Information: liter flow is dependent on which vehicle is being used to deliver the oxygen (e.g., cannula, mask, Ambu bag)

Name: oxytocin

Alias: Pitocin

Medication Class: oxytocic

Use: induces or stimulates labor; controls postpartum hemorrhage; contracts the uterus after a cesarian section

Features: given IM or IV; IV onset of action is 1 minute

Additional Information: usual adult dosage is 10 units (IV infusion is infused at 20 to 4 microunits/min)

Name: papaverine

Alias: none

Medication Class: peripheral vasodilator

Use: treats arterial spasm

Features: can be given PO, IM or IV; should not be used in patients with complete heart block; usual IM/IV dose is 30 to 120 mg every 3 hours as needed

Additional Information: none

Name: tranylcypromine

Alias: Parnate

Medication Class: MAOI, antidepressant

Use: treats depression; treats migraine headaches

Features: given PO

Additional Information: can cause blood pressure changes; usual dose is 10 mg BID

Name: Pentothal

Alias: thiopental

Medication Class: general anesthetic

Use: induces anesthesia; short-term general anesthesia

Features: given IV; onset is 30 to 40 seconds

Additional Information: usual adult induction dose is 210 to 280 mg

Name: famotidine

Alias: Pepcid

Medication Class: H_2 antagonist

Use: decreases gastric secretions

Features: can be given PO or IV; onset immediate if given IV

Additional Information: should be used with caution in children younger than 12 years; usual IV dose is 20 mg

Name: pentazocine

Alias: Talwin

Medication Class: opiate analgesic

Use: controls moderate to severe pain

Features: can be given PO, SC, IM or IV; may cause drowsiness and respiratory depression; IV onset of action 2 to 3 minutes

Additional Information: usual SC, IM or IV dose is 30 mg every 3 to 4 hours

Name: potassium chloride

Alias: KCl; K-Lor; Micro-K; Slo K

Medication Class: electrolyte

Use: prevents and treats low serum potassium levels

Features: may be given PO or IV; too much may cause cardiac arrhythmias or cardiac arrest; ECG needs to be monitored

Additional Information: usual adult IV dose is 20 mEq/hour

Name: milrinone

Alias: Primacor

Medication Class: inotropic; vasodilator

Use: treats CHF that does not respond to other medications

Features: given IV; contraindicated in the setting of acute myocardial infarction

Additional Information: usual adult dose is 50 µg/kg given as a bolus over 10 minutes followed by an infusion of 0.375 to 0.75 µg/kg/min

Name: procainamide

Alias: Pronestyl

Medication Class: antidysrhythmic

Use: treats ventricular arrhythmias

Features: given IV; should not be given to patients in severe heart block

Additional Information: usual adult dose is 25 to 50 mg/min to a total of 17 mg/kg (not to exceed 500 mg) followed by an infusion of 2 to 6 mg/min

Name: procaine

Alias: Novocaine

Medication Class: local anesthetic

Use: local and regional anesthesia including epidural, spinal and peripheral nerve block

Features: should not be used in children younger than 12 years; duration of action is 1 hour; vital signs and ECG need to be monitored throughout anesthesia

Additional Information: available in 1%, 2% and 10%

Name: protamine

Alias: none

Medication Class: heparin antagonist

Use: reverses effects of heparin

Features: given IV

Additional Information: usual dose is 1 mg protamine for every 100 U of heparin that was given (not to exceed 50 mg in 10 minutes); administer over 1 to 3 minutes

Name: pyridostigmine

Alias: Regonol

Medication Class: anticholinesterase

Use: reverses nondepolarizing muscle relaxants

Features: can be given PO, IM or IV; should not be used in patients with bradycardia or hypotension

Additional Information: usual IV dose is 10 mg to 30 mg

Name: metoclopramide

Alias: Reglan

Medication Class: cholinergic

Use: prevents nausea and vomiting; increases gastric emptying

Features: can be given PO or IV; should not be given to patients who are sensitive to procaine or procainamide

Additional Information: usual dose is 10 mg

Name: sevoflurane

Alias: Ultane

Medication Class: inhalation anesthetic

Use: inducts and maintains general anesthesia

Features: has a more rapid/smooth onset and recovery than some other gases

Additional Information: can cause bradycardia and hypotension; reduces cardiac output; may cause post-operative nausea and vomiting

Name: scopolamine patch

Alias: Transderm Scop

Medication Class: antiemetic; anticholinergic

Use: reduces nausea in patients prone to motion sickness

Features: patch delivers a dose of 0.5 mg over 72 hours; may cause dizziness or drowsiness

Additional Information: patch is placed behind the ear; not recommended for use in children; should not be used in patients with glaucoma

Name: sodium bicarbonate 8.4%

Alias: bicarb

Medication Class: alkalinizer

Use: treats documented acidosis

Features: given IV; each bristojet contains 50 mEq (50 mL)

Additional Information: usual dose is 1 mEq/kg; blood gases need to be checked frequently to avoid overalkalization

Name: succinylcholine

Alias: Anectine; Quelicin

Medication Class: depolarizing neuromuscular blocker

Use: causes skeletal muscle relaxation; facilitates intubation

Features: can be given IM or IV; onset of action is 1 minute with a duration of 6 to 10 minutes

Additional Information: should not be used in patients with a history of malignant hyperthermia

Name: terbutaline

Alias: Brethine

Medication Class: bronchodilator

Use: treats bronchospasm, asthma; stops premature labor

Features: can be given PO, SC or by inhaler; may cause tremors, palpitations and tachycardia

Additional Information: PO doses should be given with food; usual adult inhaler dose is 2 puffs every 4 to 6 hours; usual SC dose is 0.25 mg every 8 hours

Name: tetracaine

Alias: Pontocaine

Medication Class: local anesthetic

Use: used as regional anesthesia, including peripheral nerve blocks, epidural, spinal and caudal

Features: duration of action is 3 hours

Additional Information: vital signs and ECG should be monitored during anesthesia; should not be used in patients with severe liver disease

Name: theophylline

Alias: Quibron; Theolair; Uniphyl

Medication Class: spasmolytic

Use: treats bronchospasm associated with chronic obstructive pulmonary disease, asthma and bronchitis

Features: can be given PO, rectally or via IV infusion; may cause tremors, palpitations and tachycardia

Additional Information: should not be used in patients with tachyarrhythmias; usual PO dose is 100 to 200 mg every 6 hours

Name: ticlopidine

Alias: Ticlid

Medication Class: platelet aggregation inhibitor

Use: reduces the risk of stroke; can be used in patients undergoing open heart surgery

Features: given PO; increases risk of bleeding; can decrease digoxin levels in the blood

Additional Information: usual PO dose is 250 mg BID

Name: Tolinase

Alias: tolazamide

Medication Class: antidiabetic

Use: treatment of type 2 diabetes

Features: given PO

Additional Information: usual dose is 100 mg or 250 mg/day (titrated to blood sugar level)

Name: ketorolac

Alias: Toradol

Medication Class: nonsteroidal anti-inflammatory

Use: control of mild to moderate pain

Features: can be given PO, IM or IV

Additional Information: should not be used in patients with asthma or allergies to NSAIDs; usual IM/IV dose is 30 mg every 6 hours

Name: valproic acid

Alias: Depakene; Depakote

Medication Class: anticonvulsant

Use: controls seizures; controls manic episodes associated with bipolar disorder; treats migraine headaches

Features: given PO; onset of action 15 to 30 minutes

Additional Information: usual dose for migraines is 250 mg BID

Name: vancomycin

Alias: Vancocin

Medication Class: anti-infective

Use: treats organisms resistant to other antibiotics

Features: given PO or IV; overdosing can cause ototoxicity and/or nephrotoxicity

Additional Information: usual adult IV dose is 500 mg every 6 hours

Name: diazepam

Alias: Valium

Medication Class: benzodiazepine

Use: reduces anxiety; provides musculoskeletal relaxation; controls acute seizures

Features: can be given PO, IM or IV; short acting; will make patient drowsy

Additional Information: usual dose is 2 mg to 10 mg PO, lesser amounts IV

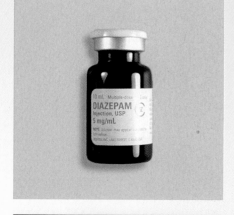

Name: vasopressin

Alias: Pitressin

Medication Class: pituitary hormone

Use: treats cardiac arrest; diabetes insipidus; bleeding esophageal varices

Features: comes 20 units per vial; need 2 vials for a dose

Additional Information: cardiac arrest dose is 40 units IV one time only

Name: vecuronium

Alias: Norcuron

Medication Class: nondepolarizing neuromuscular blocker

Use: causes skeletal muscle relaxation; facilitates intubation

Features: given IV; duration of action is 45 to 60 minutes

Additional Information: usual dosage for patients over age 9 years is 0.08 to 0.10 mg/kg

Name: verapamil

Alias: Calan

Medication Class: calcium channel blocker

Use: treats supraventricular tachycardias; treats chronic stable angina pectoris

Features: can be given PO or IV; should not be given to patients with second- or third-degree heart block, patients with CHF or patients with systolic BP <90

Additional Information: usual adult IV dose is 5 to 10 mg given over 2 minutes

Name: midazolam
Alias: Versed
Medication Class: benzodiazepine
Use: reduces anxiety preoperatively; induces conscious sedation; reduces amount needed of more potent anesthetics
Features: short acting; will make patient drowsy; twice as potent as diazepam (Valium)
Additional Information: 1 to 2 mg IV push; patient's oxygen saturation and respiratory rate must be monitored post-administration (can cause respiratory depression)

Name: Coumadin
Alias: warfarin
Medication Class: anticoagulant
Use: treats deep venous thrombosis, pulmonary embolus, acute myocardial infarction and postcardiac valve replacement
Features: given PO
Additional Information: usual dose is 10 to 15 mg/day, titrated to coagulation studies

Name: Zemuron
Alias: rocuronium
Medication Class: nondepolarizing neuromuscular blocker
Use: causes skeletal muscle relaxation; facilitates intubation
Features: given IV; duration of action about 0.5 hour
Additional Information: usual dose is 0.6 mg/kg

Name: Zofran
Alias: ondansetron
Medication Class: antiemetic
Use: prevents nausea/vomiting
Features: can be given PO or IV
Additional Information: usual adult dose is 4 mg given over 30 seconds

Name: flumazenil

Alias: Romazicon

Medication Class: benzodiazepine antagonist

Use: reverses benzodiazepines; commonly given to reverse the effects of midazolam (Versed)

Features: given IV only; compatible with normal saline, lactated Ringer's solution or dextrose in water IV solutions

Additional Information: 0.2 mg IV over 15 seconds; may be repeated in 0.2 mg doses every 60 seconds up to a maximum of 4 doses

Name: neostigmine methylsulfate

Alias: Prostigmine

Medication Class: anticholinesterase

Use: reverses nondepolarizing muscle relaxants (vecuronium, rocuronium); treats myasthenia gravis

Features: slows heart rate, thus atropine or glycopyrrolate may be given at the same time (using separate syringes)

Additional Information: usual reversal dosage is 0.5 mg to 2.0 mg IV; can be repeated as needed up to a maximum of 5 mg

Name: scopolamine hydrobromide

Alias: hyoscine

Medication Class: antiemetic; anticholinergic

Use: reduces nausea, vomiting and dizziness in patients prone to motion sickness

Features: most commonly administered via transdermal patch but can be given IV (0.4 mg)

Additional Information: not recommended for use in children; should not be used in patients with glaucoma; causes dilation of pupils

Surgical Session Review

1) The purpose of _____ is to absorb carbon dioxide in the anesthesia machine breathing circuit.
   a. soda lime
   b. limestone
   c. soap stone
   d. soda pop

2) _____ is the medication used in the treatment of malignant hyperthermia.
   a. Decadron
   b. Lasix
   c. dantrolene
   d. digoxin

3) A reading of below _____ on the BIS monitor means the patient is unconscious.
   a. 80
   b. 90
   c. 70
   d. 60

4) A _____ _____ is type of blanket that blows warm air over the patient's skin surface to help prevent hypothermia.
   a. Bear Hugger
   b. Bair Hugger
   c. Bare Hugger
   d. Bear Blanket

5) _____ is used to reverse the effects of narcotics.
   a. digoxin
   b. Decadron
   c. Narcan
   d. atropine

6) Pediatric defibrillation pads may be used on children weighing up to _____ kg.
   a. 10
   b. 15
   c. 20
   d. 30

7) The strength of epinephrine used in a cardiac arrest situation is:
   a. 1:100
   b. 1:1000
   c. 1:10,000
   d. 1:100,000

8) The strength of epinephrine used to treat an allergic reaction is:
   a. 1:100
   b. 1:1000
   c. 1:10,000
   d. 1:100,000

9) Your patient is feeling nauseated. Which of the following medications might anesthesia give to the patient?
   a. Narcan
   b. Kytril
   c. sodium bicarbonate
   d. Lidocaine

10) A setting of 2–3 liters of oxygen per minute would be an appropriate setting for a:
   a. Ambu bag
   b. nonrebreather mask
   c. oxygen mask
   d. nasal cannula

11) _____ forceps may be used during intubation to help guide the ETT.
   a. Magill
   b. Maguile
   c. DeBakey
   d. Mayo

12) Isoflurane and sevoflurane are:
   a. antiemetics
   b. antipyretics
   c. inhalation anesthetics
   d. IV anesthetics

13) _____ can be used to treat a patient with symptomatic bradycardia.
   a. Lidocaine
   b. amiodarone
   c. vasopressin
   d. atropine

14) The anesthesiologist asks for the TEE. What does TEE stand for?
   a. transesophageal endoscope
   b. transendotracheal endoscope
   c. transesophageal echocardiogram
   d. transendotracheal echocardiogram

15) When the infant's head is about to be delivered in a C-section, which of the following should you have ready to hand to the surgeon to suction the newborn's mouth and nose (assume no meconium issues)?
   a. DeLee suction
   b. Blue Bulb syringe
   c. Meconium aspirator
   d. Yankaur suction

16) A Salem Sump tube is a type of:
   a. ETT
   b. nasogastric tube
   c. wound drain
   d. suction catheter

APPENDIX

Answers to Surgical Session Reviews

ANSWERS FOR SURGICAL SESSION: CHAPTER 1

1. c
2. b
3. b
4. d
5. d
6. d
7. d
8. a
9. c
10. c
11. c
12. a
13. c
14. d
15. b
16. d
17. a
18. c
19. d
20. c

ANSWERS FOR SURGICAL SESSION: CHAPTER 2

1. a
2. b
3. c
4. d
5. b
6. a
7. d
8. b
9. a
10. b
11. c
12. d
13. a
14. c
15. c
16. b
17. c
18. a

19. c
20. d
21. b

ANSWERS FOR SURGICAL SESSION: CHAPTER 3

1. c
2. b
3. a
4. d
5. c
6. d
7. b
8. a
9. d
10. b
11. c
12. b
13. c

ANSWERS FOR SURGICAL SESSION: CHAPTER 4

1. c
2. b
3. b
4. a
5. d
6. d
7. d
8. c
9. b
10. c
11. b
12. c
13. c
14. a
15. d
16. b
17. a
18. a
19. c
20. b

ANSWERS FOR SURGICAL SESSION: CHAPTER 5

1. b
2. c
3. d
4. c
5. a
6. c
7. b
8. c
9. b
10. b
11. d
12. d
13. b
14. a
15. d
16. d
17. c
18. a
19. c
20. a

ANSWERS FOR SURGICAL SESSION: CHAPTER 6

1. c
2. d
3. c
4. b
5. d
6. b
7. a
8. c
9. d
10. c
11. c
12. d
13. a
14. d
15. b
16. c
17. c
18. b
19. c
20. b

ANSWERS FOR SURGICAL SESSION: CHAPTER 7

1. b
2. a
3. d
4. c
5. d
6. b
7. c
8. a
9. c
10. d
11. c
12. d
13. c
14. b
15. c
16. c
17. c
18. a
19. b
20. c

ANSWERS FOR SURGICAL SESSION: CHAPTER 8

1. a
2. c
3. d
4. b
5. c
6. b
7. c
8. b
9. b
10. d
11. a
12. c
13. d
14. c
15. b
16. b

Index